Continuing Professional
Development in Nursing

Continuing Professional Development in Nursing

A GUIDE FOR PRACTITIONERS AND EDUCATORS

Edited by

Francis M. Quinn

Stanley Thornes (Publishers) Ltd

First published in 1998 by:
Stanley Thornes (Publishers) Ltd
Ellenborough House
Wellington Street
CHELTENHAM
GL50 1YW
UK

ISBN 0 7487 3333 7

A catalogue record for this book is available from the British Library.

98 99 00 01 02 / 10 9 8 7 6 5 4 3 2 1

Typeset by Columns Design Ltd, Reading
Printed and bound in Great Britain
by TJ International Ltd, Padstow, Cornwall

Contents

Contributors

Christine Butterworth
Senior Lecturer, School of Post Compulsory Education and Training, University of Greenwich, London, UK

Philip Gill
Director, Quadra Consulting, London, UK

Pat Grant
Senior Lecturer in Nurse Education, School of Post Compulsory Education and Training, University of Greenwich, London, UK

Sue Hinchliff
Head of Continuing Professional Development, RCN Institute, Royal College of Nursing, London, UK

Cathy Hull
Head of Curriculum and Publishing, Macmillan Open Learning, London, UK

Christopher Maggs
Director of Research and Development and Professor of Nursing, Staffordshire University, UK

Stella Parker
Head of School of Continuing Education and Robert Peers Chair in Adult Education, University of Nottingham, Nottingham, UK

Francis M. Quinn
Director of Healthcare Education, School of Post Compulsory Education and Training, University of Greenwich, London, UK

Elizabeth Redfern
Nurse Education Consultant and lately Assistant Director for Continuing Education at the English National Board for Nursing, Midwifery and Health Visiting, London, UK

Liz Stubbings
Senior Lecturer, Nursing and Health Informatics, School of Health, University of Greenwich, London, UK

Maureen Theobald
Lately Chair, English National Board for Nursing, Midwifery and Health Visiting, London, UK

Linda Thorne
Director of Short Course Centre, School of Health, University of Greenwich, London, UK

Lynn Woodward
Senior Lecturer, Midwifery and Health Informatics, School of Health, University of Greenwich, London, UK

Preface

The professional practice of nursing, midwifery and health visiting takes place in a context of continuous change. New developments are constantly being introduced, influenced by such factors as government initiatives and improvements in medical and nursing science. Professional nurses cannot hope to practise safely and effectively unless they engage in continuing professional development (CPD) to maintain an up-to-date knowledge base to underpin that practice and to facilitate the regular and ongoing monitoring and evaluation of their own practice. Indeed, nurses, midwives and health visitors are now required to undertake CPD in order to maintain their registration with the United Kingdom Central Council for Nursing, Midwifery and Health Visiting (UKCC).

The aim of this book is to provide practitioners and educators in nursing, midwifery and health visiting with a comprehensive guide to issues and approaches in CPD, utilizing a range of contributors from both within and outside the nursing professions who possess acknowledged expertise in the field of CPD. The book covers a wide spectrum of CPD issues and approaches, and the practical 'how to do it' focus is balanced by a sound underpinning of analysis and discussion.

Following the success of our first book *Healthcare Education: The Challenge of the Market* (Humphreys and Quinn 1994), Professor John Humphreys and I conceived the idea for this new book. The original intention was that we would be joint editors, but in the meantime John was appointed vice-chancellor at the University of Greenwich.

I would like to acknowledge John's contribution, and to offer my thanks to him for our collaborative partnership across a wide range of initiatives in healthcare education. I would also like to express my sincere thanks to all the contributing authors for their chapters, to Stanley Thornes Publishers for their helpful approach, and finally to my wife Carole for the stimulating professional discussions that helped clarify my thinking for the chapters that I contributed to this book.

Francis M. Quinn
Fleet, Hampshire, UK, May 1998

Introduction: continuing professional development in nursing

1

Francis M. Quinn

In a profession that boasts some 640 000 qualified nurses and midwives registered with the UKCC (RCN, 1997), the continuing professional development of nurses constitutes a major investment. The concept itself has appeared in a number of different guises over the years, including staff development, continuing education, professional development and lifelong learning. Indeed, the contributing authors of this book by no means adopt the same term to describe what is essentially the same concept!

The aim of this introductory chapter is to 'set the scene' for the contributions that follow in the rest of the book. An overview is given of a range of issues and developments in relation to CPD in nursing, midwifery and health visiting, and this is linked to each contributing chapter.

A range of individuals and organizations can be said to have an interest in the continuing professional development of nurses (Figure 1.1), and the diagram provides a conceptual framework for this introductory chapter.

GOVERNMENT

It is axiomatic that government policy will, of necessity, impact on continuing professional development in nursing; this impact is not confined solely to Department of Health (DoH) initiatives, but includes policies emanating from other government departments such as the Department for Education and Employment. Some initiatives are targeted specifically at nurses, midwives and health visitors, whereas others have more general implications for CPD.

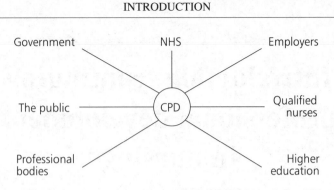

Figure 1.1 Continuing professional development in nursing: interested parties

A Vision for the Future

In *A Vision for the Future* (DoH, 1995a) five key areas and 12 targets are identified for nursing, midwifery and health visiting. Three of the targets focus directly on CPD, as follows.

- **Target 5**. Clinical and professional leaders should have taken steps to discuss with each nurse, midwife and health visitor how they might develop their practice.
- **Target 10**. Discussion should be held at local and national level on the range and appropriateness of models of clinical supervision and a report made available to the professions.
- **Target 12**. Each provider unit should be able to identify particular pre- and postregistration programmes planned to help nurses, midwives and health visitors acquire the necessary skills associated with *The Health of the Nation*, *Caring for People* and the Patient's Charter/Named Nurse initiative.

The government has acknowledged the need to update *A Vision for the Future*, and at the time of writing has announced that it will be launching a national consultation to develop a strategy for nursing, midwifery and health visiting.

Making it Happen

The importance of CPD for nurses in relation to public health is underlined in *Making it Happen* (DoH, 1995b): 'We recommend that Health Authorities should ensure that the educational opportunities available to their senior health-care personnel, including nurses, midwives and health visitors, incorporate public health aspects of commissioning and purchasing'.

The Challenges for Nursing and Midwifery in the 21st Century

The centrality of CPD in nursing is nicely captured in paragraph 112 of *The Challenges for Nursing and Midwifery in the 21st Century* (DoH, 1994): 'So a wide variety of instruments – education, training, retraining, experimentation and research – must be focused on a common objective: change within continuity. To ensure that this happens, and that nurses are released to take up their opportunities, there will need to be a common purpose shared by policy-makers at the highest level, commissioners and providers.'

There are other government initiatives that are targeted to the widest possible audience but also have implications for CPD in nursing; some are health-related, such as the Green Paper *Our Healthier Nation*, and others are education-related, such as the Fryer Report and *The Learning Age*.

Our Healthier Nation (Green Paper)

The government launched its Green Paper in February 1998 (DoH, 1998), the aims of which are as follows:

- to improve the health of the population as a whole by increasing the length of people's lives and the number of years spent free from illness;
- to improve the health of the worst off in society and to narrow the health gap.

The Green Paper is specifically focused on the health of those individuals who are worst off in society and who experience inequalities in health. This requires government action in tandem with other organizations and initiatives, such as the Food Standards Agency to reduce food-related illness; the National Minimum Wage and the New Deal to combat unemployment; initiatives to reduce crime and fear of crime; reduction of air pollution to combat respiratory illness such as asthma. Partnerships at local level between health authorities and other relevant organizations are also seen as being vital components of the proposals. Unlike the large number of targets in *The Health of the Nation*, national and local targets are set in just four areas of major ill health:

- Heart disease and stroke
- Accidents
- Cancer
- Mental health.

The Green Paper suggests four national targets to be achieved by the year 2010 in relation to these four areas:

- the death rate from heart disease, stroke and related illness in the under 65s to be reduced by at least one-third;
- accidents to be reduced by at least one-fifth;
- death rate from cancer in the under-65s to be reduced by at least one-fifth;
- death rate from suicide by at least one-sixth.

The government proposes a three-way National Contract for Health involving government, local agencies and individuals, each taking responsibility for improving health. The focus for the drive against inequalities in health will be schools, workplaces and neighbourhoods, thus covering the spectrum of age groups from children through to older individuals.

The Fryer Report

The first report of the National Advisory Group for Continuing Education and Lifelong Learning (*Learning for the 21st Century*) was published in late 1997 (DFEE, 1997), and its terms of reference were as follows.

To advise the Secretary of State on matters concerning adult learning as required, and with particular reference to extending the inclusion in lifelong and work-based learning to those groups and individuals whose increased participation will contribute to improvements in employability, regeneration, capacity building, economic efficiency, social cohesion, independent living and citizenship generally; and to make proposals in respect of:

- the preparation of a government White Paper on Lifelong Learning;
- the strengthening of family and community learning;
- the contribution of further and higher education to adult learning, having regard to relevant recommendations of the Kennedy Committee on widening participation in FE and the National Committee of Inquiry into the future of HE;
- initiatives for development in the context of the University for Industry;
- the development of Learning Towns and Cities.

Clearly, there are implications for the nursing and midwifery professions arising out of the report, since it is aimed at all sections of society. The report highlights the lack of a lifelong learning culture in the UK and the fact that education and training are considered inadequate to meet competitive challenges. According to the report, only 14% of employees participate in job-related training, while one-third say they have never been offered such training by their employer.

The report proposes a ten-point agenda for the development of a lifelong learning culture, as shown in Figure 1.2.

Section 10 of the report focuses on promoting lifelong learning at the workplace, which includes:

- job-related learning, i.e. specific learning to improve job performance;
- transferable-skills learning, i.e. to produce a more responsive and flexible workforce;
- personal development learning, i.e. knowledge and skills to help people make employment or career changes and to facilitate their personal fulfilment.

In February 1998, the government downgraded its lifelong learning plan from a White Paper to a Green (consultation) Paper, and this was published as *The Learning Age: a Renaissance for a New Britain* (DFEE, 1998a).

1. Development of a strategic framework for the promotion of lifelong learning.
2. A campaign to revolutionize attitudes to lifelong learning.
3. A commitment to widening participation and achievement in learning.
4. Increased emphasis on home, community and workplace as places of learning.
5. A need for simplification and integration of qualifications and learning pathways.
6. Development of effective partnerships, planning and collaboration to provide lifelong learning opportunities for all.
7. Provision of information, advice and guidance for people to access lifelong learning and to begin to take some responsibility for developing their own learning.
8. A need for new data, targets and standards to underpin the new strategy.
9. Effective use of the new technologies of communication and information to support lifelong learning.
10. A need to ensure that funding and finance stimulate a far wider group of participants and do not constitute barriers to lifelong learning.

Figure 1.2 Ten-point agenda for lifelong learning

The Learning Age: A Renaissance for a New Britain

While no direct reference is made within the Green Paper to continuing professional development, the document has implications for everyone: 'Learning is the key to prosperity – for each of us as individuals, as well as for the nation as a whole. To realise our ambition, we must all develop and sustain a regard for learning at whatever age.' Within the Green Paper, the government acknowledges the Fryer Report's call for the development of a new culture of lifelong learning, and identifies the benefits for individuals, businesses, communities and the nation.

The paper sets out a number of initiatives through which the government's strategy for lifelong learning will be carried forward. The references to the Dearing Report are included in the section on higher education later in this chapter; the key points of the Green Paper are outlined below.

University for Industry (UfI)

The University for Industry 'will act as the hub of a brand new learning network, using modern communication technologies to link businesses and individuals to cost-effective, accessible and flexible education and training'. The UfI will provide information and advice about courses via enquiry desks in towns, telephone, fax, e-mail and web site. As well as delivering learning packages to individuals' homes through a variety of media, the UfI will have learning centres to which its students can go to access courses and materials. These learning centres will be operated by a wide range of providers, including further education colleges, universities and private sector institutions, and the UfI will be backed up by extensive advertising and publicity.

Learning Direct

This is a new national helpline to provide free, confidential, impartial and up-to-date information about the availability of provision, and can link the individual with a range of agencies such as further education, higher education and private sector providers.

Individual learning accounts

This is a national system, the aim of which is to provide an incentive for adults to undertake training. It is based on the principles that (1) investing in learning is a shared responsibility and (2) the individual is in the best position to decide what and how s/he needs to learn. The accounts will be available to all and will enable individuals to save and borrow to invest in their own learning. Following consultation, a framework will be constructed for the delivery of individual learning accounts.

Learning at work

The Green Paper highlights the variable spread and quality of training in the workplace and the need for workplaces to become centres of learning; this will be encouraged by a legislative framework. Investors in People will become the standard for staff development in both public and private sectors, and a National Skills Task Force will be established to assess future skill needs, strengthen partnerships at local level, disseminate information on changing skill needs, and tackle skill shortages in collaboration with other agencies such as the new employer-led National Training Organizations (NTO).

In 1997 the English National Board for Nursing, Midwifery and Health Visiting was awarded a grant from the European Commission that supported an international symposium on raising the quality of health service provision through the development of lifelong learning. This culminated in a report entitled *Lifelong Learning in Europe: Developing a Strategic Approach.*

In Chapter 3, Sue Hinchliff discusses lifelong learning in nursing.

THE NATIONAL HEALTH SERVICE

The NHS sector still employs some three-fifths of registered nurses, but there has been a significant increase in the numbers of such nurses in the non-NHS sector and in GP practices. However, recruitment to all sectors is currently showing a shortfall, due in part to a reduction in the numbers of nurses being trained. The Royal College of Nursing points out that large numbers of nurses will retire in the next 5 years, adding to the recruitment problem beyond the millennium (RCN, 1997).

In Chapter 5, Philip Gill explores the role of professional development in workforce planning for the NHS.

Changes within the NHS sector inevitably have a knock-on effect on CPD for nurses. In 1997 the government produced a White Paper on the new NHS that has important implications for CPD in nursing, midwifery and health visiting (DoH, 1997).

The New NHS *(government White Paper)*

The White Paper introduces primary care groups into the NHS to replace the system of general practitioner (GP) fundholding by 1999; these groups will consist of GPs and community nurses, who together will be responsible for commissioning primary health care and are accountable to health authorities by means of annual accountability agreements. Primary care groups will each have a governing body representing general practice, community nursing and social services, and will include public involvement; greater recognition is given to the role of community health councils. The White Paper also emphasizes public health, with health authorities being given a greater strategic role in the assessment and planning of health improvement programmes for local populations. The Patient's Charter will be replaced by a more comprehensive NHS charter, and a 24-hour telephone advice line, staffed by nurses and called NHS Direct, will be set up to provide information and advice; this should help ease overcrowding in GP surgeries and accident and emergency departments.

Two new quality bodies will be created, the National Institute for Clinical Excellence and a statutory body, the Commission for Health Improvement. The former will focus on clinical and cost effectiveness, including clinical audit; the latter's role is to offer an independent guarantee that local monitoring systems are in place to ensure and improve the quality of clinical services.

Clinical audit

Monitoring of quality is a vital aspect of the health service, mediated through initiatives such as clinical audit and Health Services Accreditation.

Clinical audit or patient care audit 'provides an opportunity for professionals who provide health-care services to work together to set standards for services to patients, to measure their actual practice against the standards, and to make improvements in service as indicated' (NHS Training Directorate, 1994). It provides the opportunity to transform the quality of services; at the time of writing, initiatives are under way to bring together the strands of clinical audit (currently being done separately by medical practitioners, nurses, and other health professionals) into a unified multiprofessional clinical audit system. A good example of a CPD resource is the NHS Training Directorate's facilitator's guide for trainers who are involved in teaching other staff how to implement clinical audit.

Health Services Accreditation

The aim of Health Services Accreditation is 'to act as an effective, continuous improvement mechanism for quality in the National Health Service' (Health Services Accreditation, 1997). The unit is managed by a consortium of health authorities on a non-profit-making basis, and the system involves three stages.

1. **Accreditation standards**. These consist of guidelines for service providers on the minimum levels of service to be achieved, plus examples of good practice.
2. **Accreditation**. Accreditation instruments, in the form of a series of questions, are used to identify the type of evidence required to demonstrate the achievement of standards. Accreditation visitors are independent specialists drawn from the health-care professions.
3. **Reporting of results**. This stage involves the reporting of the results to both the service provider and the health authority; the former then has targets for the future and the latter has independent evidence of quality.

The Health Service Accreditation Unit also publishes a quarterly magazine, *The Standard,* which is distributed free to professionals responsible for quality management.

Information management and technology

Information management and technology (IM & T) is now a familiar resource in most areas of the NHS. Nursing practitioners need to be familiar with the principles and use of such technology, so it is important that CPD is made available for those practitioners who lack the basic knowledge, skills and experience in this medium. The Education and Training Programme in Information Management and Technology has commissioned an assessment and resource indicator pack for IM & T across nursing curricula (Education and Training Programme, 1997). The pack is part of the Enabling People programme and is designed to support teachers in the implementation of IM & T in their curricula. The pack contains six units, which include audit and quality, workload and skill mix, information technology, information synthesis and presentation, and contracting. The pack adopts a needs identification approach combined with a range of resources to meet those needs.

In Chapter 12, Liz Stubbings and Lynn Woodward address the field of nursing informatics.

EMPLOYERS

Although the majority of registered nurses are employed within the NHS, there were some 50 000 whole-time equivalent (WTE) nurses working in the non-NHS sector in 1997 (RCN, 1997). CPD for nurses is an important element in the maintenance of standards of delivery of care in both sectors, but it can also be used as a marketing strategy to indicate a quality organization. For example, some private nursing homes employ only first-level registered nurses, and this fact is used in marketing material as an indicator of high-quality service.

THE PUBLIC

Members of the general public should have more than a passing interest in the continuing professional development of nurses, given that we are all potential patients or clients of the health-care industry. Although they may be unfamiliar with the concept of CPD, the public have certain expectations about the nurses who care for them; for example, they expect them to have up-to-date knowledge and skills appropriate to the specialism in which they practise, and also that they demonstrate a thoughtful and caring approach in their dealings with them and with their nearest and dearest.

People are generally much more informed about health matters than previous generations have been, mainly because of the growth of media interest in all aspects of health. However, the downside to this is the phenomenal growth of 'therapists' of all kinds, from colour therapists to cinema therapists. The public have a right to be safeguarded against malpractice by nurses or other practitioners, and to be protected from charlatans. For the former, CPD may help to reduce episodes of malpractice, while professional disciplinary processes can deal with the worst-case scenario. For the latter, entry to professions can be restricted to persons of appropriate character by means of an act of Parliament or a royal charter, as is the case with nurses and physiotherapists respectively.

In 1997 the UKCC changed its rules to allow the Professional Conduct Committee to remove from the register, for a specified period of time, any nurse found guilty of professional misconduct. Such practitioners would, at the expiry of that time, have to apply for the restoration of her/his name to the register. The UKCC has the power to reject applications for restoration if it believes that an offence is incompatible with registration as a nurse. 'The UKCC is determined to uphold public faith and confidence in the good name of the nursing, midwifery and health visiting professions' (UKCC, 1997a). The UKCC has now been given approval to implement a rule change allowing nurses found guilty of serious disciplinary offences to be struck off the register for fixed minimum periods.

In Chapter 6, Maureen Theobald explores the concept of monitoring to keep the patient safe.

QUALIFIED NURSES

The motivation to undertake continuing professional development by nurses may arise from a range of different needs. The most obvious one that springs to mind is the UKCC's PREP requirements, to which all registered nurses must conform if they are to continue on the register of nurses. There are also more altruistic motives, such as a desire to improve the standard of practice, and other less altruistic ones, such as gaining further qualifications to enhance promotion prospects or a desire to increase personal status by the acquisition of bachelor's, master's or doctoral degrees. There is even the possibility that some nurses may see CPD as providing evidence of safe practice in cases of litigation by patients or clients.

A great many qualified practitioners can be classified as postregistration students, as they are pursuing formal courses as part of their CPD. For the majority of these nurses, their studies will be undertaken while they are in full-time employment. The position with regard to study leave and funding for CPD has worsened considerably in the recent past, and the best that they can expect to obtain is partial funding; study leave to attend formal courses is even more difficult to obtain and in cases where it is granted, the demands of service mean that it may not always be possible to take it. Hence, the demand for more flexible approaches to study has led to the development of open and distance learning programmes which allow postregistration students to study in their own time and without the need for attendance at an institution (a case study of one such distance learning programme for nurse teachers is included later in this chapter).

Another significant development in the delivery of CPD for nurses is the accreditation of prior learning (APEL); this has enabled experienced practitioners to identify learning gained within the workplace, to provide evidence of such learning in a portfolio and to use the credit thus gained to contribute towards the final award. For many nurses, this has meant a considerable reduction in the amount of time taken to gain a higher education award.

In Chapter 11, Christine Butterworth and Linda Thorne explore the accreditation of prior learning.

PROFESSIONAL BODIES

It could be argued that, in some shape or form, continuing professional development in nursing has always happened – for example, by reading relevant professional journals, attendance at postregistration courses such as those of the now-defunct Joint Board of Clinical Nursing Studies (JBCNS), statutory courses such as lifting and handling, the ENB's 'refresher' courses for nurse teachers, and the important area of on-the-job training. The current position, however, is dramatically different, in that CPD is now a requirement for continuing registration, in the form of the UKCC's PREP requirements.

In Chapter 2, Christopher Maggs explores the contribution that a philosophy of continuing education can make to nursing.

The United Kingdom Central Council for Nursing, Midwifery and Health Visiting (UKCC)

The UKCC Code of Professional Conduct (UKCC, 1992a) states that registered nurses, midwives and health visitors are required:

to act, at all times, in such a manner as to:

- safeguard and promote the interests of individual patients and clients;
- serve the interests of society;
- justify public trust and confidence; and
- uphold and enhance the good standing and reputation of the professions.

Continuing professional development has a major role to play in maintaining this requirement, and paragraph 3 of the Code specifically relates to CPD: 'maintain and improve your professional knowledge and competence'. The importance of CPD is further underlined in paragraph 3 of *The Scope of Professional Practice* (UKCC, 1992b):

Foundation education alone, however, cannot effectively meet the changing and complex demands of the range of modern health care. Post registration education equips practitioners with additional and more specialist skills necessary to meet the special needs of patients and clients.

In its paper *Issues Arising From Professional Conduct Complaints* (UKCC, 1996a), the UKCC identifies an agenda for action; under 'issues for management' it emphasizes the importance of support and supervision for practitioners. The issue of supervision is also addressed in the UKCC's *Position Statement on Clinical Supervision for Nursing and Health Visiting* (UKCC, 1996b).

In Chapter 8, Pat Grant and Francis M. Quinn discuss clinical supervision in nursing.

The most significant development relating to CPD in nursing is the UKCC's requirements for postregistration education and practice (PREP).

PREP is about developing individual nurses, midwives and health visitors in order to maintain and improve standards of patient and client care. PREP enables you to maintain and improve the standard of knowledge and competence which you have achieved at the point of registration in order to promote higher standards of practice. (UKCC, 1977b)

As part of the PREP requirements, every practitioner must undertake a minimum of 5 days or equivalent of study activity every 3 years, and also maintain a personal professional profile containing details of professional development.

It is interesting to contrast this compulsory form of CPD with the self-monitoring system adopted by the Chartered Society of Physiotherapy. The Society defines CPD as 'the educational process by which professional people maintain, enhance and broaden their professional competence' (CSP, 1995), and recognizes that 'the concept of lifelong learning is an essential pre-requisite to maintaining clinical competence'. There are 11 standards for CPD that every physiotherapist must undertake, as indicated in Figure 1.3.

---

1. Reflection on practice through self-evaluation
2. Recording of ongoing CPD activity
3. Identification of ongoing requirements for CPD
4. Contacting professional bodies/professionals/professional groups for assistance in planning CPD
5. Planning CPD with line manager
6. For physiotherapists who work single-handedly, planning CPD with support from other physiotherapists
7. Selection of activities for CPD that enhance professional competence
8. Evaluation of whether ongoing objectives of CPD are met
9. Liaison on a regular basis with the manager concerning evaluation of CPD, which is an integral part of the annual performance appraisal
10. For single-handed practitioners, evaluation with a peer group of whether the objectives of CPD have been met
11. Sharing of knowledge and skills with other practitioners

Figure 1.3 Standards for CPD (CSP, 1995)

The Society has also developed a self-audit tool for practitioners to use in the monitoring of their ongoing CPD programmes.

In Chapter 3, Sue Hinchliff discusses in detail the UKCC PREP requirements. In Chapter 9, Liz Redfern explores the personal professional profile. In Chapter 7, Francis M. Quinn discusses reflection and reflective practice in nursing.

The English National Board for Nursing, Midwifery and Health Visiting

In 1992 the ENB Framework and Higher Award for continuing professional education for nurses, midwives and health visitors came into operation, and aims to assist practitioners to develop the knowledge and skills necessary to meet the changing needs of the population. The framework is a partnership between practitioners, managers and educationalists, and there are five stages to be considered when a practitioner commences it.

1. **Review**. The practitioner reviews his/her expertise and achievements with his/her current client group in relation to the key characteristics, and index for the Higher Award if desired.
2. **Contract**. With the collaboration of the manager, a contract is entered into with the educational institution to identify learning outcomes for the award.
3. **Delivery**. The practitioner then participates in the educational activities to achieve the learning outcomes, including maintaining an individual professional portfolio.
4. **Assessment**. Achievement of learning outcomes is demonstrated by assessment and recorded in the portfolio.

5. **Quality assurance**. Practitioners, educationalists and managers will review the relevance and effectiveness of the learning experiences undertaken.

Ten key characteristics are identified as representing the knowledge, skills and expertise necessary for the provision of quality care to meet changing health needs, and the integration of all these can be recognized by the Higher Award. This is at a minimum of first-degree level and requires demonstration of mastery of the ten key characteristics into a field of professional practice. The ten key characteristics are given in Figure 1.4.

1. Professional accountability and responsibility
2. Clinical expertise with a specific client group
3. Using research to plan, implement and evaluate strategies to improve care
4. Team working and building, multidisciplinary team leadership
5. Flexible and innovative approaches to care
6. Use of health promotion strategies
7. Facilitating and assessing development in others
8. Handling information and making informed clinical decisions
9. Setting standards and evaluating quality of care
10. Instigating, managing and evaluating clinical change

Figure 1.4 The ten key characteristics (ENB, 1991)

The outcomes for the Higher Award can be achieved through a range of activities such as in-service courses, open learning, self-instruction, and taught courses. Practitioners working towards the Higher Award are required to maintain a personal professional portfolio.

There are similarities between the ENB Framework and Higher Award and the UKCC's PREP standards, and the Board sees the former as providing a firm foundation for the latter's implementation (ENB, 1995). The Board has taken action to implement the UKCC's transitional arrangements for use of the title 'specialist practitioner'; a number of institutions have been approved to undertake the assessment of practitioners' portfolios of certificated learning against the learning outcomes of an ENB recordable course. The Board has also approved large numbers of specialist practitioner programmes, some two-thirds of which are in the community area and the remaining one-third in the acute area (ENB, 1997).

The National Board for Nursing, Midwifery and Health Visiting for Northern Ireland

The National Board for Nursing, Midwifery and Health Visiting for Northern Ireland (NBNI) has had a distinctive education role in comparison with the other three national boards, in that it owned the four colleges of nursing within the province and employed the teaching staff within those colleges. In 1997 this unique arrangement ceased when the four colleges of nursing were incorporated into the Queen's University of Belfast. This section describes the NBNI's Continuing Education Framework, the aims of which are stated as follows:

> The Continuing Education Framework is directed toward assuring the quality of nursing and midwifery care by preparing practitioners to:
>
> - plan and deliver nursing care to high standards and levels of excellence;
> - assess quality and evaluate care;
> - take appropriate action to ensure that the quality of care is developed and improved within available resources;
> - participate with managers, other professionals and clients in an overall approach to care delivery which assures quality and the most cost-effective use of resources.

The framework reflects the principles of career-wide development, standardization, flexibility, and credit accumulation and transfer, and consists of three stages.

- **Stage 1** is concerned with consolidation of competence following registration for all practitioners, and is normally in the practitioner's current field of practice. This stage would also meet the requirements for return to practice, and the study units are at CATS level 2.
- **Stage 2** is designed to meet the UKCC PREP standards for practitioners who wish to work in the areas of specialist practice, education, research and management. The level of study must be not less than first-degree level.
- **Stage 3** aims to prepare practitioners for senior managerial or advisory roles, and the level of study is set at CATS level 3 and may also include master's level.

HIGHER EDUCATION

The higher education (HE) sector is a key player in the continuing professional development of nurses, being the main provider of academic awards. CPD generates business for HE institutions, and the increasing demand for flexible CPD provision has helped stimulate interest in open and distance learning, and accreditation of prior learning.

The Dearing Report

The Dearing Report (*Higher Education in the Learning Society. Report of the National Committee of Inquiry into Higher Education*) was published in summer 1997, and its terms of reference were:

> to make recommendations on how the purposes, shape, structure, size and funding of higher education, including support for students, should develop to meet the needs of the United Kingdom over the next 20 years, recognis-

ing that higher education embraces teaching, learning, scholarship and research. (Dearing, 1997)

This very comprehensive report makes 93 recommendations, a number of which have important implications for the continuing professional development of both practitioners and teachers of nursing.

Recommendations 9, 13, 14, 15, 47 and 48 refer specifically to staff development, and three main aspects are covered:

- the need for institutions to review, update and make available to all staff their policies with regard to staff development;
- the need for institutions to review the impact of communications and information technology on the role of staff, and ensure that the necessary support and training is made available;
- that an Institute for Learning and Teaching in Higher Education (ILT) should be established for the purpose of accrediting programmes of teacher training, the commissioning of research into teaching and learning, and the encouragement of innovation. All new full-time academic staff should undertake ILT-accredited teacher training as part of their probationary period of employment.

Recommendation 22 and Executive Summary points 42–45 focus on a proposed framework for higher education qualifications. The framework consists of eight levels, as shown in Figure 1.5.

H1. Certificate
H2. Diploma
H3. Bachelor's degree
H4. Honours degree
H5. Higher honours/postgraduate conversion diploma
H6. Master's degree
H7. MPhil
H8. Doctorate

Figure 1.5 Framework for higher education qualifications

The proposed framework includes both academic and vocational qualifications and provides for progression through the whole range of achievement. It also embraces credit accumulation and credit transfer between institutions, and each level in the framework must have recognized standards.

The English National Board for Nursing, Midwifery and Health Visiting (ENB) has responded in detail to the Dearing Report, identifying issues that have implications for the education of nurses, midwives and health visitors (ENB, 1998). With regard to the third recommendation above, on teaching qualifications, the Board expressed the view that 'programmes should lead to recognised qualifications in teaching at the appropriate academic level instead of merely consisting of short modules for developing a range of skills'. The response also emphasized that preregistration nursing and midwifery education should remain in the higher education sector rather than further education, given that it is at degree level. Since continuing professional development also occurs at master's and doctoral level, a split of provision between the two sectors is not appropriate.

The Board also expressed concern about recommendation 34, that institutions should consider whether they wish to enter departments in the next Research Assessment Exercise, or alternatively to seek lower-level, non-competitive funding for research to underpin teaching. This potential separation of universities into research- or teaching-only, the Board maintains, would jeopardize the progress made in nursing research over recent years.

Higher Education for the 21st Century

In February 1998 the government published its response to the Dearing Report (DFEE, 1998b). This section of the chapter will address the response to the recommendations relating to staff development that were highlighted in the previous section.

The government welcomed the recommendations on the need for institutions to review and update their staff development policies and to make these available to staff, and encouraged institutions to follow up these recommendations. They also welcomed the recommendations on the need for training and support of both staff and students in communications and information technology, and identified the importance of the Institute for Learning and Teaching (ILT) in the endorsing and development of these materials. With regard to the recommendations concerning the ILT, the government states that the Institute will be established by September 1998; its functions should be the accreditation of programmes of training for HE teachers, the commissioning of research and development into effective teaching and learning practice, and the stimulation of innovation. The issue of accredited teacher training is also welcomed:

> the Government's long-term aim is to see all teachers in higher education carry a professional qualification, achieved by meeting demanding standards of teaching and supervisory competence through accredited learning or experience.

The government also considers that one way of improving the quality of teaching is to make available examples of outstanding teaching, on film, video or by broadcasting, and will invite the ILT to consider setting up a national system for this.

The Dearing recommendations with respect to a framework for higher education qualifications are endorsed by the government, particularly the need for a national credit accumulation and transfer (CAT) system and the introduction of more, separately accredited 'stopping-off points' to enable students to assemble the 'building blocks' of qualifications.

In Chapter 4, Stella Parker explores continuing professional development in the context of adult and higher education.

Distance learning and open learning

Although the origins of flexible learning can be traced as far back as the turn of the
century in the work of writers such as John Dewey, the humanistic educational culture of the 1960s and 1970s provided the real thrust for its further development.
The writings of Carl Rogers on client-centred therapy, and its corollary, student-
centred learning, emphasized the pre-eminence of student empowerment and
autonomy, and these ideas found fertile soil in those educators wishing for a more
humanistic approach to teaching and learning. During this period there was also a
growing interest in the opening up of access to further and higher education using
alternatives to traditional entry qualifications, and also flexible methods of delivery. The best known British example of a mass, open-access, distance learning
scheme originating at this time is the Open University.

In addition to these general factors, the 1980s found nurse education experi-
encing severe resource constraints on continuing professional education, with
employers placing limitations on the amount of funding available for attendance
at courses, and reduced opportunities for study leave. The creation of the NHS
internal market gave employers a much greater say in the kind of continuing education provision they required for their nursing staff, including more flexible
approaches to course delivery. Humphreys and Quinn (1994) concluded that the
orthodox curriculum paradigm that characterizes nurse education is increasingly
incompatible with the requirements of the market, and proposed a new curriculum
paradigm to replace it

In Chapter 10, Cathy Hull discusses the approach to open learning adopted by
Macmillan Open Learning.

Distance learning can be defined as follows:

> Distance Learning, also called Distance Education, is an educational deliv-
> ery system that is planned on the basis of wide geographical separation of
> educational provider and student, and utilising textual materials and other
> media such as radio and television broadcasts, videotapes, telephone and
> computer communication. (Quinn, 1995)

The following case study illustrates a distance learning approach to initial
teacher training at the University of Greenwich.

CASE STUDY: THE UNIVERSITY OF GREENWICH POSTGRADUATE CERTIFICATE IN EDUCATION (PGCE) BY DISTANCE LEARNING

This multiprofessional, in-service programme provides initial teacher training for
teachers in the postcompulsory sector, and is approved by the English National
Board for Nursing, Midwifery and Health Visiting for recording as a teacher of
nurses and midwives on the register of the UKCC.

The development of a more flexible approach to initial teacher training in this postcompulsory sector of education followed extensive market research, which identified three principal factors affecting provision: declining resources, the increasingly effective in-house provision by client colleges and the sustained pace of curriculum and organization change within the sector (Land and Humphreys, 1994). Many potential students are prevented from undertaking in-service teacher training because they are unable to obtain day-release to attend courses, and even if they manage to obtain day-release this may often clash with departmental meetings and other employment-related demands.

Hence, the provision of a distance learning mode offers a flexible alternative that allows the student to study at times convenient to her/him and obviates the need for attendance except for the occasional workshop session once or twice a year.

The distance learning programme consists of core and option units delivered in the form of printed distance learning materials and augmented by tutorial support from a named personal tutor. The latter is also responsible for carrying out observation and assessment of the student's teaching performance within the student's educational employment setting. Tutor/student contact is maintained by telephone, letter, fax and e-mail, the main method being dictated by the availability of appropriate media to the student.

Within the last two years a new aspect of communication has been introduced to the programme, computer-mediated tutoring, which is defined as 'the use of computers, telephone lines and specialist software to facilitate interaction between students and tutors irrespective of geographical location or time zone' (Ryan, 1996). This system uses Lotus Notes to offer both electronic mail and conferencing databases; e-mail can be used for one-to-one messages and questions or for one-to-many notices and information. Computer conferencing allows students and tutors to discuss issues in a 'virtual group', but does not take place in real time. Hence, a tutor may initiate activities or introduce ideas on to the server and the students in the virtual group can respond at any time of the day or night. Students and tutor may initiate and respond to each other's inputs just like a live seminar, but with the advantage of not having to be in the same place at the same time.

The implementation of distance learning has a number of operational implications, e.g. the availability of tutors outside the normal working day. Most students undertake this type of programme because they are fully committed to their employment during the working day. There is therefore little point in offering a tutorial service between the hours of 09.00 and 17.00; rather, the students will want tutorial contact in the evenings or at weekends. To operate such a system requires a fundamental rethink of tutorial staff timetables if overloading is to be avoided. Ideally, distance learning tutors should deal exclusively with such programmes, to avoid conflict with teaching times on attended courses.

Access to distance learning programmes is another issue: since flexible provision implies that educational provision should be available when the student wants it, this presents a challenge to institutional systems, e.g. the scheduling of examination boards. Tutorial support is another challenge: institutions often use tutors who live close to distant students so as to facilitate tutoring, and this can present difficulties in ensuring that they maintain good communication with the institution, and also in their attendance at staff development activities.

As one would expect, there are both costs and savings in the use of distance learning, and these need to be weighed carefully when considering implementation. The greatest cost is the development and production of the distance learning materials: an editorial board is required; writers need to be commissioned; decisions about design and quality of the materials will influence cost; critical readers need to be commissioned; materials need to be piloted – all of which have very substantial cost implications. Materials will not remain up to date for ever and so review and updating will need to be scheduled every 3–5 years depending upon the nature of the materials. There are also costs involved in the necessary staff development for distance learning tutors.

There are, however, some potential savings from the implementation of distance learning. For example, it is possible to make savings on the use of paper materials by downloading the units on to the students' computers. In comparison with attended courses, distance learning does not require classroom space nor is there a need for face-to-face class contact between teachers and students, both of which consume considerable resources. Also, by freeing up the tutors from heavy class contact, there may be more time available for staff to undertake research, an increasingly important issue in the light of the Research Assessment Exercise. The use of high-quality textual and computer material can be a far more effective learning strategy than poorly delivered lectures, and from a quality assurance point of view is much more open to public scrutiny than the latter.

REFERENCES

CSP (1995) *Standards for Continuing Professional Development (CPD)*, Chartered Society of Physiotherapy, London.
Dearing, R. (1997) *Higher Education in the Learning Society*. Report of the National Committee of Inquiry into Higher Education, HMSO, Norwich.
DFEE (1997) *National Advisory Group for Continuing Education and Lifelong Learning for the 21st Century* (document reference: PP62/31326/1197/43), Department for Education and Employment, London.
DFEE (1998a) *The Learning Age: a Renaissance for a New Britain* (Green Paper), Stationery Office, London.
DFEE (1998b) *Higher Education for the 21st Century, Response to the Dearing Report*, Stationery Office, London.
DoH (1994) *The Challenges for Nursing and Midwifery in the 21st Century, The Heathrow Debate*, Department of Health, London.
DoH (1995a) *A Vision for the Future*, NHS Management Executive, Leeds.
DoH (1995b) *Making it Happen. Public Health – The Contribution, Role and Development*

of Nurses, Midwives and Health Visitors, Report of the Standing Nursing and Midwifery Advisory Committee, Department of Health, London.

DoH (1997) *The New NHS* (White Paper), HMSO, London.

DoH (1998) *Our Healthier Nation* (Green Paper), Stationery Office, London.

Education and Training Programme (1997) *ADAPT for Teaching and Learning: An Assessment and Resource Indicator Pack for IM & T across nursing curricula*, Enabling People Programme, Solihull.

ENB (1991) *Framework for Continuing Professional Education for Nurses, Midwives and Health Visitors: a Guide to Implementation*, English National Board for Nursing, Midwifery and Health Visiting, London

ENB (1995) *The Future of Professional Practice: the Board's Response to PREP*, English National Board for Nursing, Midwifery and Health Visiting, London.

ENB (1997) *Annual Report 1996–1997*, English National Board for Nursing, Midwifery and Health Visiting, London

ENB (1998) The Board's response to the Dearing Report. *ENB News*, **Jan**.

Health Services Accreditation (1977) *Health Services Accreditation – A Guide to the Process*, Health Services Accreditation, East Sussex.

Humphreys, J. and Quinn, F. M. (1994) *Healthcare Education: The Challenge of the Market*, Chapman & Hall, London.

Land, R. and Humphreys, J. (1994) Marketing professional development in education, in *Healthcare Education: The Challenge of the Market*, (eds J. Humphreys and F. M. Quinn), Chapman & Hall, London.

NHS Training Directorate (1994) *Getting Ahead With Clinical Audit: a facilitator's guide*, NHS Training Directorate, Bristol.

Quinn, F. M. (1995) *The Principles and Practice of Nurse Education*, 3rd edn, Stanley Thornes, Cheltenham.

RCN (1997) *Factsheet 4* (Sept.), Royal College of Nursing, London.

Ryan, M. (1996) Using computer-mediated communication to support distance learners, *EHE Evaluation Report 89*, University of Greenwich, London.

UKCC (1992a) *Code of Professional Conduct for the Nurse, Midwife and Health Visitor*, 3rd edn, United Kingdom Central Council for Nursing, Midwifery and Health Visiting, London.

UKCC (1992b) *The Scope of Professional Practice*, United Kingdom Central Council for Nursing, Midwifery and Health Visiting, London.

UKCC (1996a) *Issues Arising From Professional Conduct Complaints*, United Kingdom Central Council for Nursing, Midwifery and Health Visiting, London.

UKCC (1996b) *Position Statement on Clinical Supervision for Nursing and Health Visiting*, United Kingdom Central Council for Nursing, Midwifery and Health Visiting, London.

UKCC (1997a) Protecting the public, protecting the good name of our professions. *UKCC Register*, **Autumn**.

UKCC (1997b) *PREP and You*, United Kingdom Central Council for Nursing, Midwifery and Health Visiting, London.

A philosophy of continuing professional education in nursing

2

Christopher Maggs

INTRODUCTION

This paper explores the contribution a philosophy of continuing professional education makes to nursing and examines the characteristics of such a philosophy. In order to do so, the paper looks at what is meant by continuing professional education (CPE) and the current issues that create the demand for CPE. It describes the approach taken to attempt the construction of a philosophy of continuing professional education, rejects the idea that such a philosophy is desirable and then goes on to outline the key values that must be present if CPE is to underpin practice.

BACKGROUND

Change is commonplace in human affairs but what cause anxiety or apprehension in people are the pace of change and the feeling of being out of control. Nowhere is this felt more strongly than in the health-care system and in those professions, like nursing, that are at the hub of change. These tensions are felt directly in clinical practice and indirectly as a result of developments in nurse education.

The demand for new skills and abilities to improve clinical practice has a knock-on effect on the standards of continuing education and the ways in which it can be delivered. Participation in continuing education has been the subject of much research (see, for example, Rogers *et al.*, 1986) and there were in the past reports of relatively low levels of participation, particularly for specific groups like practice nurses (Rogers *et al.*, 1986). Participation rates no longer seem to be an issue and the subject of research. The statutory requirement to maintain and develop competence that is embodied in the UKCC regulations appears to have been a major factor in driving up the numbers attending courses. Each new development, most recently clinical supervision, clinical effectiveness and evidence-based practice, brings with it a call for education and training and there is no shortage of response from education providers.

Competition within higher education, coupled with the integration of professional and academic education, is also adding to the availability and uptake of continuing education, with educational technology developments like open and distance learning playing an increasing role in flexible access for busy working professionals.

A brief overview of the literature on CPE is instructive. As has been noted, participation seems to be less discussed than hitherto, but there are other issues to which CPE has been linked that also seem not to be as important as once thought. For example, throughout the late 1980s much attention was given to the links between effective CPE and recruitment and retention policies (Maggs, 1996; IMS, 1987). This was in part a reaction to the anticipated demographic shifts that were confidently expected to reduce the numbers of 18-year-olds available for work. Whatever the impact of the demographic change and whenever it will be felt within health care, the fact remains that linking CPE to recruitment and retention policies is not high on the agenda for many NHS trusts and employers. Indeed, despite a renewed anxiety about future recruitment, the previous almost inseparable link between CPE and recruitment and retention no longer seems to exist.

Perhaps what has happened is that fewer and fewer people – practitioners, managers, employers – need to be persuaded of the benefits of CPE to service developments and that it is now axiomatic that service development is always associated with CPE. The most prominent issue now is not the need to justify CPE but the ability to pay for it in a resource-limited system. The introduction of education consortia that purchase pre- and postregistration education and training on behalf of NHS trusts may well drive up 'quality' but drive down 'quantity'. If, as is supposed, these bodies develop the sophistication needed to match CPE to service needs (and, therefore, to patient care), it is to be expected that they will determine, in broad terms, who does participate and in what, and should ensure a closer 'fit' between CPE and practice. The role of education consortia, at first unsophisticated but increasingly market-driven and questioning of the relevance of much continuing education to the work of NHS trusts, will have far-reaching effects not only on the amount of CPE 'purchased' but on its quality. There will, inevitably, be conflict between providers of education, mainly the university and higher education sector, and the consortia, many of which appear to be distancing themselves from the concerns and input of the universities and their nurse educators.

One consequence of the separation of purchaser and provider in CPE has been the development over time of an almost 'mechanistic' approach to CPE and programmes. The notion of 'utility' has crept in by the back door, as employers and nurses seek out educational opportunities that are said to have direct relevance to the role or post. A quick glance through job advertisements will confirm this anec-dote. Specific CPE qualifications are tied to particular grades or roles and, increas-ingly, this means possession of a degree in or relevant to nursing. Again, despite the interest of the English National Board in evaluating programmes, there remains little systematic evidence of the 'fit' between qualifications and hence CPE and roles and duties in clinical practice.

There is, therefore. a need to address the nature of that 'fit' and how CPE will underpin and ensure effective clinical practice. There ought not to be any argument about the responsibility of the individual to maintain and develop the appropriate knowledge, skills and expertise required for the care s/he provides. This is the essence of the UKCC requirements for continuing registration. There is likely to be little dispute about the importance of focusing CPE on the needs of patients and clients for clinically effective nursing care. There may be debate about how these are linked and articulating a philosophy of continuing professional education pro-vides one way of demonstrating that they should be. If there were such a statement, which was informed by the range of values and beliefs of all those concerned – patients, nurses, managers, etc. – it would have practical and strategic implications for nurses, teachers and the health service (Maggs, 1996; Bailey, 1988).

DEVELOPING A PHILOSOPHY OF CPE: THE EXPERT GROUP

A large-scale project was undertaken in the early 1990s by the English National Board for Nursing, Midwifery and Health Visiting (ENB) to devise a new frame-work for CPE for the nursing and midwifery professions. It was recognized that, in addition to the many other aspects that required rethinking, the absence of an articulated philosophy of CPE was a major inhibiting factor in its development. It was also felt that the body charged with the statutory duty of approving pro-grammes in postregistration education should state its approach to and its set of values for continuing professional education.

Under the direction of the project manager, a group of experts was brought together to debate the issues surrounding CPE and to work towards creating a set of values or beliefs which the ENB could use to drive forward its framework for CPE.

The members of the expert group included teachers, practitioners, health ser-vice managers, experts in CPE from other professions and an ethicist.

The group met formally over two whole days, with a one-day follow-up meet-ing after a draft had been written up. The method of working was a mixture of large-group work, in which participants made statements that were then debated, and small discussion groups, which served to flesh out the details of some of the broad statements agreed in the plenary sessions. Each large-group meeting was chaired by the project manager and the small groups nominated one member to act as chair and to report back to the whole group. Regular resumés of progress were given and, at the end of the first day, a summary of agreements and disagreements was drafted to prepare members for the second day's work.

The first session was given over to a discussion about the purpose of the group, which exposed two key issues that coloured the rest of the debates. Firstly, most members felt that the group could devise a set of belief statements but not 'a philosophy' of CPE and, secondly, the group argued that, having done so, the profession should 'own' it. In other words, the statement of the set of beliefs had to be made public and not solely used 'in-house' to guide curriculum or policy development. The debate was wide-ranging on both issues and became, at times, quite heated. This was a salutary lesson for all present because it betrayed the passion and importance attached to linking CPE and practice for the benefits of patients and clients in the health service.

On the question of a set of beliefs or a philosophy, the group felt that it was important to spell out in some detail why they thought that their task was to devise a set of belief statements and not a philosophy. In discussion, it was argued that individuals might well hold or subscribe to specific philosophical principles that might be different.

For example, one person might hold that the fetus had a right to life that was unequivocal and that no exceptions could be permitted, while another might hold that no such right existed and that therefore abortion was permitted. Both could be nurses and act morally while not sharing the same philosophical principle. To try and reach agreement on a single philosophical stance on CPE was, the group felt, both impossible and undesirable.

The expert group also agreed that individuals who belong to a particular collective entity, e.g. a profession, do hold in common certain values and beliefs that distinguish them from another collective entity. For example, nurses agree on the value of respect for their patients, irrespective of their views about the status of the fetus. Patients can expect that nurses will treat them with respect at all times and nurses have an obligation to do so at all times. These collective values and beliefs are constructs of the profession and entrants to and members of the profession acquire them (if they do not already share them) through professionalization, which includes professional education and practice.

Debating beliefs and a belief system

It was agreed, therefore, to concentrate the energy of the group on exploring shared values and beliefs and working towards producing an agreed statement to encapsulate them. The group defined a belief system as 'a series of beliefs and values which provide a framework for action through a set of principles' (Maggs, 1996). For the purposes of CPE, therefore, a belief system of education was seen as a second-order statement of beliefs, values and principles derived from those philosophical principles that inform people's actions as individuals and as members of a profession, in this case nursing.

The philosophical principles that characterize the profession of nursing are supported by a belief system for education which ensures that those professional principles are attained and maintained. Education is the operationalizing of the fundamental philosophical principles that underpin the profession and the belief system of education will be one that engenders and sustains the professional role.

There should be, it follows, a belief system of nursing, derived from first principles, that forms the basis of the professional relationship. This, together with the general beliefs and values held by the individual and the belief system of education, provides the framework for the policies and practices of CPE in nursing.

The values of nursing

The group next turned their attention to the core values of nursing, derived from first principles. In discussion, a number of statements of the values of nursing were explored and common elements were identified. Nursing, it was suggested, focuses on assessing the health needs of people, providing assistance to them when they are ill or need help, and supporting them as they work towards self-care and take back responsibility for their health (MSDGH, 1995). Midwifery shares these essentials but focuses primarily on working with mothers in a natural, non-medical way to ensure a healthy pregnancy and a healthy child (MSDGH, 1995). As a consequence, the group adopted the following statement of the purpose of nursing as a guide to its work on a belief system for CPE:

> The goals or purposes of nursing include support for people during the activities and events of life, from birth to death, using skills, strengths and knowledge to enable people to maintain their own balance of health, and assisting them in illness and disability towards greater understanding and return to autonomy or, at the end of life, to a dignified death. (Riverside, undated)

The group recognized that there were any number of statements already made about the philosophy of nursing but felt that the Riverside Health Authority statement of purpose encapsulated those philosophies in a way that made sense to practitioners and encapsulated the views of the expert group itself.

Personal values and belief systems

The group finally sought to clarify what it meant by personal values and beliefs, given their focus on nurses as professionals. The expert group agreed that a personal belief system provides individuals with the means of expressing their values, understanding their world and locating their place in it. It is a guide to action and a way of others knowing what to expect from the individual. It is intensely personal, based on the uniqueness of the individual, and a way of helping to maintain the individual's autonomy and integrity.

Personal belief systems are under constant challenge from the belief systems of others, new events and novel experiences. The personal belief system is incremental, interactive and unfolding or else it loses its humanity.

There is a continual tension between being and becoming – individuals reach landmarks and objectives but, in so doing, open up new, previously unknown challenges, opportunities and experiences (Passmore, 1970). The process of challenge and change is a maturing process, one which should be dynamic, dialectic and potential (Passmore, 1970).

Continuing professional education: a definition

The next stage of the process was to agree what was meant by continuing professional education. Whatever the definition, and there are several, all accept that CPE is an essential characteristic of a profession. CPE may be limited to formal courses leading to postregistration qualifications or maintaining them. It might be seen as part of career development or the development of the profession as a whole. There is general agreement that, whatever its operational purposes, it is, indeed, 'continuing' and lasts throughout the individual's personal and professional career.

The group discussion ranged over many of the key issues to do with CPE and lifelong learning, including accountability and responsibility; the relationship between education and training; the ways in which knowledge and skills can build on previous levels of expertise and expertness; and the moral 'imperative' to maintain and develop competence and confidence. It was also agreed that the personal and the professional were in symbiotic relationship, itself a creative and educational experience.

Of equal importance is the acknowledgement that the professional relationship between nurse and patient should, through reflection in and on practice, be a learning experience (Downie and Telfer, 1987).

Continual reappraisal of that relationship, built upon the value systems within the nursing therapeutic relationship, provides opportunity for personal and professional growth.

Following the debate, the definition that was adopted for the purposes of constructing a belief system of CPE was as follows:

> CPE is a term used to encompass those teaching and learning activities, including open and experiential learning, which follow registration and are directed at improving the quality of care provided to the public. CPE experiences develop the habit of lifelong learning, by which the individual practitioner, the profession and the health service are able to critically evaluate quality of care and implement research outcomes in practice. (Maggs, 1996)

Continuing professional education: a belief system

The group concluded that a belief system of continuing education in the nursing and midwifery professions:

> recognises each practitioner as an autonomous person whose professional goal is to instigate, sustain and develop the professional relationship

between nurse and patient within an agreed belief system of nursing.
(Maggs, 1996, p. 100)

That statement includes the recognition that the nurse has a wider existence as a member of society, with many and changing roles which inform the way the nurse acts as nurse. Snow and Willard (1989) have drawn attention to the negative consequences of the integration of nurse and person roles, where the person roles may be unresolved conflicts of long standing (they argue, for example, that the origins of such conflicts that spill into professional life and behaviour lie in 'child abuse (anything that shames a child)') and where the nurse uses nursing and caring as a 'veil' for the outfalls from the unresolved conflicts. The positive aspect needs to be celebrated but must first of all be explored. In other words, the interdependence of the personal and the professional is not a given but is itself a creative, experiential and educative act.

It is also the case that CPE is about 'adulthood' and not the education of a child. This in turn argues for taking a high and developed degree of personal and individual responsibility for actions and experiences, including professional CPE. It also means that responsibility cannot be delegated to another, especially an employer. However, it is possible that the exercise of personal responsibility will involve, for most nurses, working with and through an employer to obtain the best outcome for professional development. The employing authority, in meeting its contractual and statutory duties, should endeavour to provide appropriate opportunities for the individual practitioner to maintain and develop skills, knowledge and expertise in nursing.

The definition includes experiential learning and argues that this is both professional and personal. Professional experiential learning may come through supervised practice followed by reflection or exposure to new and challenging practice situations that are discussed in a supportive peer relationship. Unless there is some notion of either reflection or 'assessment' of these new clinical experiences, no matter how 'informal' these may be, there can be little evidence of learning in the sense of accountability.

While experiential learning in and through practice may be demonstrated, experiential learning in non-professional roles may be more difficult to establish as relevant to practice and as a learning event.

A schematic approach, in which outcomes of experiential learning in non-professional settings are set against professional practices, may be one way forward. For example, personal experience of bereavement and grief can lead to greater insights into the needs of carers and relatives in similar situations, as can the experience of motherhood support professional skills in communication or developing relationships. Obviously, not everyone who experiences bereavement can or may wish to 'translate' that experience into the professional arena. The important issue is that the nurse should have the opportunity to examine experiences in non-professional roles and to learn from them, where appropriate. Given the earlier comment about the integration of the personal and the professional, this approach to experiential learning seemed to the group to be incontrovertible.

Perhaps of most importance, the definition clearly addresses the need for the research base to practice and the links that must be forged between CPE and outcomes of nursing interventions. This laudable aim, however, has to be set within the context of the degree to which such research-based evidence exists and the extent to which it has meaning for the nurse and for the curriculum for CPE events.

Reflections on the development of the belief system of continuing professional education

Given the paucity of debate about a philosophy of continuing professional education in nursing and midwifery (in contrast to the literature on CPE in the medical profession – see the ground-breaking works of Cyril Houle (1980), for example), it might be suggested that such a statement is unnecessary. It might be the case, as is argued here, that a philosophy is an illusion but that a belief system is not.

It might also feel uncomfortable in the British context to have to have such discussion and debate – after all, there is a dearth of philosophers of nursing who are British and speak to the British culture: There may be those who will wish to criticize the way in which this project went about its task and therefore challenge its conclusions. This final section reflects on these and other issues and attempts to overcome any shortcomings that may appear to exist in the foregoing description of a belief system of continuing professional education in nursing and midwifery.

TOWARDS A BELIEF SYSTEM OF CPE: THE WAY OF WORKING

First, let us dispose of the criticisms, if any are raised, of the way in which the conclusions presented here were reached. The group was a highly selective group with no notion of representation nor mandate from interest groups. The discussion and debate, while informed, were personal. Conflicting opinion cannot be reflected in what is necessarily a consensus statement, as here. There is no record of the proceedings, other than the printed document or article.

Seeking a consensus statement from a group in which members may hold many views demands, I would suggest, as much rigour as might be associated with more empirical research. The role of the convenor, moderator, facilitator or chairperson is a key factor in establishing and maintaining that rigour. Debate, as in this case, was the essential characteristic of the way of working and debate, by its nature, can become heated. What should transpire, in the well-managed group, is a learning process in which the views of members are challenged and altered or reinforced, depending on the arguments put forward. Statements of fact are assessed for 'confidence' and applicability, statements of opinion 'tested' against 'evidence'.

More usefully, a process of 'multiple triangulation' should occur. In such an expert group, each discipline present points its concepts and conclusions at the others, and all focus on the issue to hand. Where even the language used by one discipline may be unfamiliar to another, each seeks to establish common ground.

Testing the degree of consensus can be carried out quite simply by providing feedback to members and inviting their comments on the content. This requires that the chairperson or facilitator maintains a degree of impartiality and independence from the group and its deliberations, something which may more easily be wished for than achieved.

Why is CPE necessary?

The self-evident fact that nursing practice and nursing science are evolving phenomena is a powerful argument for continuing professional education. While controversy may rage about the nature of nursing practice and science, what nurses do and how they behave in everyday clinical situations demands ongoing education. Skills development as well as the maintenance of existing competence are clearly justifications in themselves for CPE.

We should also, perhaps, be moving away from the instrumentalist, mechanistic and reductionist associations between CPE and management strategies, including recruitment and retention and even service development, and towards a view that CPE is, in itself, the way in which the art and science of nursing are created, challenged and sustained. This would have much more resonance with preregistration education, through which the 'novice' enters the world of professional knowledge, skill and expertise. It is not a necessary reason for the development of a graduate profession but a graduate profession would seem a sufficient condition for CPE to provide that role in nursing science.

How does CPE link to practice?

It might well be that the question is not whether CPE is necessary but what form it should take. Alternative educational approaches, like open and distance learning, accreditation of prior or experiential learning, have been around for some time and are well discussed in the literature. Before making decisions about the 'technology', it is useful to explore briefly what CPE seeks to address.

There is a current trend, stimulated by the introduction of evidence-based medicine (EBM; Sackett et al., 1997) towards the implementation of evidence-based practice (EBP) and evidenced-based nursing (EBN; Cullum et al., 1997). This innovation has been generated, in part, by the belief that not only is there a plethora of new treatments in health care, medicine and in nursing, but that there are 'new types of evidence which, when we know and understand them, create frequent, major changes in the way that we care for our patients' (Sackett et al., 1997, p. 6). Evidence-based practice offers, it is claimed, the opportunity of addressing clinical problems through rigorous selection of 'best available evidence', from sources such as randomized controlled trials (RCTs), systematic reviews and meta-analyses, and from primary research, and applying those findings in the clinical situation. A hierarchy of evidence is suggested, with RCTs at the top and non-randomized and small-scale studies much lower down.

According to some of its protagonists, especially but not uniquely Sackett *et al.* (1997), there are also major flaws in the way in which clinicians access information created in this new way. Numerous explanations, reasons and excuses are offered for this inability to access appropriate, relevant and up-to-date information, including lack of time to read journals and the failure of many of those who have responsibility for helping clinicians to learn 'on the job', in practice, to keep up to date themselves (Sackett *et al.*, 1997, pp. 8–9).

What EBM claims to offer is a different way of achieving the goals of CPE through a new form of practice, EBM. Pointing to the growing evidence for tenuous links between practice and continuing medical education (CME), Sackett *et al.* (1997) argue that 'traditional, instrumental CME simply fails to modify our clinical performance and is ineffective in improving the health outcomes of our patients' (Sackett *et al.*, 1997, p. 10). Following an RCT among medical clinicians, they conclude that 'CME and other strategies for Continuing Professional Development that employ just instructional approaches consumed by volunteers do not address the problems of our declining clinical competence' (pp. 11–12).

The answer, it transpires, is to inculcate a sense of lifelong learning based on EBM, either as the way in which professional life begins or 'through journal clubs and less traditional, active programmes of continuing professional development' (Sackett *et al.*, 1997, p. 12). This must be supplemented by a willing acceptance of the need to find and use EBM generated by others and the use of clinical guidelines and protocols developed by others using the highest possible levels of evidence.

Much but not all of what Sackett *et al.* argue for in medicine is now argued for in nursing (Cullum *et al.*, 1997). Those who follow Sackett and other medical colleagues along this road point, *inter alia*, to the paucity of the knowledge base on which nursing practice can depend, the failure to implement the findings of research into practice, and the wide variations in practice (see, for example, Cullum *et al.*, 1997).

The same criticisms that are offered against EBM may, therefore, be offered against EBN (White, 1997), not least its reductionist nature (Maggs, 1996; Jacobson *et al.*, 1997); its failure to celebrate reflective practice; its avoidance of the importance of expert intuition (Benner, 1984); and its lack of resonance with nursing science.

Any approach to CPE in nursing based primarily on EBN, *vide* EBM, will suffer from the same problems. The most important of these is that CPE in the 'new order' must be EBN-driven (see above). This pushes the dynamic and dialectic of practice and science, which includes the personal and the historical as well as the biomedical, off the board and replaces them with a single focus on the biomedical approach to health and illness (Jacobson *et al.*, 1997).

What educational approach best fits the link with practice?

We must begin by recognizing an obvious but overlooked fact of nursing life – nursing is not a hospital-based discipline but one that covers all facets and settings of human existence.

The dominance of hospital-based medicine has, historically, led to the dominance of hospital-based nursing, whatever attempts there might be to devise a primary-care-led NHS (Maggs, 1985). This is not a given but is subject to challenge and should be. Then we have to recognize that nursing is not a cold, unemotional occupation but one in which humour, sadness, uncertainty and respect for others by nurses and by patients find expression in and through the art of nursing practice.

We share, I believe, much in common, in this respect, with general practice (Jacobson *et al.*, 1997; Balint, 1957; RGCP, 1996), which Jacobson *et al.* (1997) describe as combining 'a rational, scientific method and a less rigorous "art"' (p. 451). They go on to argue that the 'art of medicine is founded upon context, anecdote, patient stories of illness, and personal experiences' (p.451). Where I might differ is the assertion that nursing science is anything other than this 'art' and that the technico-rational (which, after all, is really technological and not science) supports the art of nursing practice, which is inseparable from science as 'praxis'. If we reflect back on the definition of CPE and the belief system that generates it (described above), we can, I argue, show how this approach to CPE 'fits' best with nursing practice.

CONCLUDING REMARKS

The conventional approach to discussions about the curriculum assume that what is under debate is a course or programme of teaching and learning. There is clearly the need for such events to be designed, using the best in teaching and learning strategies and technologies.

There is another sense in which the curriculum for CPE in nursing and midwifery is a statement about the totality or wholeness of the lifelong ongoing development of the practitioner – it is a statement about the nature of nursing and about the role of the nurse. Taking such an approach is not possible in the absence of an *a priori* understanding and acceptance of fundamental principles of nursing science and values. In arguing for those values and for their expression through a system of belief of CPE, I am, I suggest, advocating a continuing demand for the articulation of a philosophy of nursing. Without that, we are lost and lack both wisdom and learning (Jacobson *et al.*, 1997, p. 451).

REFERENCES

Bailey, C. (1988) Lifelong education and liberal education. *Journal of Philosophy of Education*, **22**(1).

Balint, M. (1957) *The Doctor, His Patient and The Illness*, Pitman, London.

Benner, P. (1984) *From Novice to Expert: Excellence and Power in Clinical Nursing Practice*, Addison-Wesley, Menlo Park, CA.

Cullum, N., DiCenso, A. and Ciliska, D. (1997) Evidence-based nursing: an introduction. *Evidence-Based Nursing*, **Pilot issue**, iv–v.

Downie, R. S. and Telfer, B. (1987) *Caring and Curing: a Philosophy of Medicine and Social Work*, Methuen, London.

Houle, C. (1980) *Continuing Learning in the Professions*, Jossey-Bass, London

IMS (1987) *Attitudes, Jobs and Mobility of Qualified Nurses*, Institute of Manpower Studies, Brighton.

Jacobson, L., Edwards, A., G. and Butler, C. (1997) Evidence-based medicine and general practice. *British Journal of General Practice*, **47**, 449–452

Maggs, C. (1985) *Origins of General Nursing*, Croom Helm, London.

Maggs, C. (1996) Towards a philosophy of continuing professional education in nursing. *Nurse Education Today*, **16**, 98–102.

MSDGH (1995) *A Statement of Values in Nursing*, Mid Staffs Genera! Hospitals NHS Trust, Stafford.

Passmore, J. (1970) *The Perfectibility of Man*, Duckworth, London.

Riverside Health Authority (undated) *Philosophy for Nursing*, Riverside Health Authority, London.

Rogers, J., Lawrence, J. and Maggs, C. (1986) Evaluation of the use of distance learning materials in continuing professional education for nurses, midwives and health visitors. Unpublished report to the Department of Health.

RCGP (1996) *The Nature of General Medicine Practice. Report from General Practitioner Practice Number 27*, Royal College of General Practitioners, London.

Sackett, D., Richardson, S. W., Rosenberg, W. *et al.* (1997) *Evidence Based Medicine: How to Practice and Teach EBM*, Churchill Livingstone, Edinburgh.

Snow, C. and Willard, D. (1989) *I'm Dying to Take Care of You: nurses and codependence*, Professional Counselor Books, Redmond, USA.

White, S. (1997) Evidence-based practice and nursing: the new panacea? *British Journal of Nursing*, **6**(3), 179.

FURTHER READING

American Nurses' Association (1984) *Standards for Continuing Education in Nursing*, American Nurses' Association, Kansas City, KS.

Cervero, R. M. and Scanlan, C. L. (eds) (1985) *Problems and Prospects in Continuing Professional Education*, Jossey-Bass, London.

Confederation of British Industries (CBI) (1989) *Keeping to our Competitive Edge – The Needs for Britain to Respond to Change*, CBI, London.

Cooper, S., S. and Hombath, S. (1973) *Continuing Nurse Education*, McGraw-Hill, London.

Curtin, L. and Flaherty, M. J. (eds) (1982) *Nursing Ethics: Theories and Pragmatic*, Prentice-Hall, London.

Department of Health (1988) *The Way Ahead 1988. Report to the NHS Management Board by the Department of Health Nursing Division, Career Development Project Group*, Department of Health, London.

Department of Health (1989) *Working for Patients: Education and Training Workshop Working Paper 10*, Department of Health, London.

Department of Health Nursing Division (1988) *Strategy for Nursing*, Department of Health, London.

Duberly, J. (1985) Continuing education: whose responsibility? *Professional Nurse*, **1**, 4–6.

English National Board for Nursing, Midwifery and Health Visiting (ENB) (1992) *Framework for Continuing Professional Education and Training*, ENB, London.

Freidson, B. (1970) *Profession of Medicine: a Study of the Sociology of Applied Knowledge*, Dodd, Mead, London.

Goodland, S. (ed.) (1984) *Education for the Professions: Quid Custodiet?* SRHEE & NFER-Nelson, London.

Harnett, E. (1988) Does higher education have aims? *Journal of Philosophy of Education*, **22**(2).

Prigigione, I. and Stengers, I. (1984) *Order out of Chaos: Man's New Dialogue with Nature*, Fontana, London.

Royal College of Nursing (RCN) (1987) *In Pursuit of Excellence: A Position Statement in Nursing*, RCN, London.

Schon, D. (1983) *The Reflective Practitioner*, Basic Books, New York.

Schon, D. (1987) *Educating the Reflective Practitioner*, Jossey-Bass, San Francisco, CA.

Squires, P. (1987) *The Curriculum Beyond School*, Hodder & Stoughton, London.

Tschudin, V. (1986) *Ethics in Nursing: The Caring Relationship*, Heinemann, London.

UKCC (1984) *Code of Professional Conduct for the Nurse, Midwife and Health Visitor*, United Kingdom Central Council for Nursing, Midwifery and Health Visiting, London.

UKCC (1987) *Project 200: a New Preparation for Practice*, United Kingdom Central Council for Nursing, Midwifery and Health Visiting, London

UKCC (1989) *Information on Post Registration Education and Practice Project*, United Kingdom Central Council for Nursing, Midwifery and Health Visiting, London

Wain, K. (1987) *Philosophy of Lifelong Education*, Croom Helm, London.

3 Lifelong learning in context

Sue Hinchliff

This chapter will start by examining what is meant by lifelong learning and the values on which it is based, together with the skills and competences that support it. It will explore what makes continuing professional development effective and the importance of it being set within a culture that welcomes what it can offer. The second part of the chapter narrows the focus to examine the role of the UKCC in formally introducing lifelong learning into nursing. It will look at the long gestation period for PREP, analysing what shaped the final proposals and how they were received by the profession. The chapter will conclude by examining the North American experience of mandatory professional updating and what we can learn from this.

INTRODUCTION

'Lifelong learning' is the term often used to refer to the learning that occurs throughout the (usually working) life of an individual, which may be planned or not. Increasingly, in the late 1980s and 1990s, in further and higher education in the UK, learning arising from experience, and reflection in and on practice, has come to be recognized as a valid component of an individual's education and is given formal recognition in the accreditation of prior experiential learning (APEL).

The concept of lifelong learning acknowledges that we are in an era of continuous change and that this requires continuous learning with an acceptance of education occurring at all points in the lifespan. This implies, of course, that teaching methods appropriate to adult learners must be used, focusing on learning derived from experience, using a student-centred, needs-based approach. This – termed

andragogy (see later) – allows the learner to set his/her own agenda and assess its
success. It stresses active rather than passive learning, frequently using peers as a
source of knowledge.

The rapid pace of change in the nature of work in the latter decades of the present century necessitates both planned learning opportunities and valuing the learning that accrues from carrying out the job and reflecting on outcomes, and this is
particularly apparent in nursing.

> The growth of knowledge and increasing research in all areas of health care,
> together with the development of new technology, means that old knowledge
> and skills are no longer appropriate. (Hinchliff, 1994)

Lifelong learning can be seen, therefore, as a desirable politico-economic activity, necessary to maintain a skilled workforce in a constantly changing world.

Lifelong learning, almost by definition, is associated with liberal-democratic
and humanistic values (Knapper and Cropley, 1991) and outcomes such as:

- equality of opportunity
- the importance of self-fulfilment
- freedom to learn
- responsibility for self
- valuing what other learners can teach
- an enquiring mind, able to think critically
- facilitation rather than dictation.

are frequently expressed within this educational arena. It refers to a continuum of
learning opportunities from the formal taught mode through experiential and
reflective learning to thinking-in-action.

THE SKILLS AND COMPETENCES ON WHICH LIFELONG
LEARNING IS BASED

For lifelong learning to be a reality and effective the learner needs to work towards
achieving some prerequisite skills, and the author suggests the following, based on
a framework offered by Cropley (1981).

- **An ability to set and work towards realistic goals that are achievable
  within the constraints of the individual's personal and professional life**.
  This demands a self-directed approach towards learning. Jarvis (1987) alludes
  to the lack of information that we have in nursing about the extent of self-direction
  among nurses. However, it could be argued that a considerable degree of self-
  direction must exist in the profession, since over 44 000 applications for Royal
  College of Nursing continuing education initiatives had been made in the 2-year
  period leading up to the time when the requirements of the United Kingdom
  Central Council for Nursing, Midwifery and Health Visiting (UKCC) for
  professional updating became mandatory, on 1 April 1995. Acquisition of

evidence of professional updating, prior to this point, was not compulsory, yet nurses sought to maintain and enhance their knowledge without apparent pressure being exerted by outside influences.

Additionally, learners may need help in setting and adjusting short-, medium- and long-term goals for their own development that are realistic for them. In the author's experience mature nurse learners undertaking higher or continuing education have a tendency, initially, to attempt to aim for alpha grades when beta is more achievable (bearing in mind the demands of, say, a full-time job as a community nurse, two small children, a partner and a home to run, as well as overseeing elderly parents and in-laws and maintaining some semblance of a social life!).

- **Effective application of theory in practice to tackle work-based problems and an ability to measure the results**. New work-based problems arise as practice constantly changes, reflecting what today might be called the needs of the market. For example, with a shorter inpatient stay people are being discharged home needing different sorts of care from community nurses to that required in the past. Similarly, with the growth in day surgery, nursing care planning has had to be adapted to the restricted patient stay and standard care plans developed. Practitioners need to be able to reframe, in Handy's (1989) expression, in order to look at problems and their solutions in different ways, 'sideways or upside down: to put them in another perspective or another context: to think of them as opportunities not problems' (p. 52).

- **Maintaining motivation to learn continuously and an ability to evaluate the effectiveness of this learning**. Houle (1980) points out that 'the extent of the desire of an individual to learn ultimately controls the amount and kind of education he or she undertakes' (p. 124). He then goes on to divide practitioners into four main groups, dependent on what he calls their 'zest for learning':

  - *innovators:* a small but highly active group, who constantly seek to improve their job performance; they try out untested ideas, constantly consume educational opportunities and enjoy independent learning and full-time study;
  - *pacesetters:* not usually the first to try out new ideas, but strongly committed to professional ideals and continuing education;
  - *middle majority*: the bulk of practitioners, whose attitudes to continuing education vary from enthusiasm to apathy;
  - *laggards:* those who do the minimum necessary, resisting both learning and new ideas.

  Houle cites a fifth group, whom he called *facilitators*, comprising those who no longer actively practise, consisting of academics, editors, writers and executives, each of whom can fall into any of the preceding four groupings in terms of their motivation towards continuing their education.

- **Familiarity with a variety of learning and assessment strategies in a range of settings.** By definition this demands good study skills (see below) and a knowledge of one's own learning style. If, as said earlier, adults learn best with an andragogical approach, then the philosophy underlying this may need to be explained, since it may not accord with learners' expectations. Adults tend to learn best when:

- they experience a 'need to know' and participate voluntarily in the search for knowledge and skills to meet their perceived deficit;
- they are in an environment that is both physically and psychologically comfortable, with respect for their own worth and that of others;
- they are able to set their own goals for their achievements;
- they share responsibility for both planning and operationalizing their learning, and there is a collaborative approach;
- they engage in active rather than passive learning;
- they are encouraged to relate what they learn to their own experience, and conversely to use this experience to enrich and inform their learning;
- they feel a sense of responsibility – a sense of ownership – for their own progress.

While we know, from the work of Knowles (1984) and Brookfield (1986) and others, that adults learn best when these conditions are met, nevertheless, adults who undertook their initial school and nurse education when there was an emphasis on the teacher imparting knowledge to the learner may need space to refocus, learning that it is desirable and permissible to value that which has been derived from experience, to set goals and to see education as a collaborative partnership between teacher and learner.

- **An ability to locate relevant information and resources, using appropriate media**. If self-direction in learning is to be encouraged throughout the professional's life, then teaching study skills appropriate to this is essential. Such skills were seldom taught in the past. It is becoming more common nowadays, however, for study skills to be taught not only during schooling, but also as part of preregistration nurse education. These would include active reading, listening, problem-solving and decision-making skills, keyboard and word-processing skills, accessing information from databases, the Internet or CD-ROM, library-searching, etc. There are, however, large numbers of practitioners who were educated before this formed part of the curriculum and who trained in nursing when these skills were not taught, and so there is considerable unmet need in this area.

If we accept that the above are relevant prerequisite skills and competences, then effective programmes offering continuing professional development should focus on fostering these needs.

CONTINUING PROFESSIONAL DEVELOPMENT (CPD)

Lifelong learning embraces the linkage of education and work – the application of learning to practice and the notion that practice itself is not static. Alongside this is the acceptance that not only does theory inform a professional's practice but knowledge can also be embedded in and emerge from that practice (Schon, 1983).

In *The Scope of Professional Practice* (UKCC, 1992), the UKCC states: 'Just as practice must remain dynamic, sensitive, relevant and responsive to the changing needs of patients and clients, so too must education for practice.'

Dynamic, changing practice is underpinned by education that is work-focused. Practitioners need to be able to access knowledge and skills and develop attitudes to upgrade, consciously, systematically and continuously, their existing repertoire.

Continuing professional development – CPD (or continuing education – CE) is a way of meeting this need for education 'on the job'. The former term is preferred by the author, with its emphasis on meeting **professional** needs. It is also the term used by the majority of other professions and so is widely understood. Note that it is not intended to enter the debate about whether nursing is or is not a profession. That debate is aired eloquently elsewhere (e.g. Davies, 1995; Lorentzon, 1991; Jolley, 1989). For the purposes of this chapter, nursing is assumed to be a profession. Thus, the following definition is suggested as being appropriate to the context of nursing:

> CPD is the maintenance and enhancement of the knowledge, expertise and competence of professionals throughout their careers according to a plan formulated with regard to the needs of the professional, the employer, the profession and society. (Madden and Mitchell, 1993)

The definition finds favour on a number of counts.

- It refers both to maintaining a steady state (i.e. not entering into decline) and also to improving existing abilities.
- It suggests that CPD is about extending both knowledge and skills, and it also acknowledges the existence of expertise on the part of professionals.
- It takes a lifelong learning approach, suggesting that CPD is a career-long process.
- It implies the existence of a plan to direct this development – in line with current thinking in nursing on portfolios, profiles and individual performance review.
- It suggests that CPD is based not simply on the needs of the individual professional but also those of the employer, the profession as a whole and society. This latter – 'society' - must, for nurses, represent not only the wider population who have potential health needs but also their actual client group.

Madden and Mitchell's definition can be compared with Professor Graeme Davies's minimalist definition of continuing education (Davies, 1984) as 'training for adults which is not continuous with initial full-time education', which is somewhat bald and less helpful, with its emphasis on 'training' rather than 'education'.

Some professions use the term 'continuing professional education', which was described by an expert panel in the USA as:

the varied modes and content of education and learning that are recognised by appropriate authorities as contributing to the knowledge, competence, development and performance of individual professionals after they have been licensed as practitioners. (Hunt, 1992, p. 5)

The American Nurses' Association offered, in 1984, a definition of continuing professional education appropriate to nursing, which distinguished it from in-service training and staff development:

planned educational activities intended to build upon the educational and experiential bases of the professional nurse for the enhancement of practice, education, administration, research or theory development to the end of improving the health of the public.

The author would feel more in harmony with this definition if there were some indication that the individual who is consuming these activities had some hand in planning them. There is, however, reference to the practitioner's experiential knowledge – and presumably skills – and the range of areas to be bettered is clear and broad.

It is worth noting, however, that Jarvis (1984) suggests that the term 'continuing learning' is more acceptable than 'continuing education', since the latter smacks of courses supplied for the practitioner to attend, rather than encouraging a view of keeping abreast that encompasses reading and self-directed learning as well as attending conferences. This latter view is, of course, more in line with the notion of lifelong learning.

Madden and Mitchell's definition, however, would seem to fit most closely with the UKCC's view of what education and practice following registration is all about. The UKCC (1990) see CPD as fulfilling three functions:

(a) updating and extending the professional's knowledge and skills on new developments and new areas of practice – to ensure continuing competence in the current job;
(b) training for new responsibilities and for a changing role ... developing new areas of competence in preparation for a more senior post;
(c) developing personal and professional effectiveness and increasing job satisfaction.

In nursing we might also add that CPD is potentially a key tool in maintaining standards. Todd (1985) argues that CPD must affect practice, extending the professional's knowledge base, the actions that potentially develop from that (performance) and the effective application of what is known.

Lifelong learning is complemented by lifelong education and this refers to planned educational opportunities. Clearly, for a lifelong learner to access such planned opportunities a degree of motivation must exist. Houle (1980) argues that such a commitment to extending learning must be inculcated during initial professional preparation. Indeed, he goes as far as to suggest that:

some attention should presumably be given in the admissions process to the selection of individuals who have already given evidence that they have a thirst for knowledge and that they are likely to retain that thirst throughout their careers. (p. 82)

This is a theme that recurs in the document in which UKCC set out its plans for redesigning initial nurse education (UKCC, 1986):

we are convinced that the old tradition of a once and for all training, encyclopaedic in its objectives, cut off from other sectors and closely tied to the practice context, must be replaced. It must be replaced by a sound foundation, followed by a series of building blocks directly allied to perceived needs. The building blocks should be capable of easy modification and replacement as new needs become apparent. (p. 20)

They foresaw the emergence of 'a new animal to be regulated': 'a mature and confident practitioner, willing to accept responsibility, able to think analytically and flexibly, able to recognize a need for further preparation and willing to engage in self-development' (p. 33) and acknowledged that '[t]he programme of preparation ... will bring the practitioner to a point of safe and competent practice at registration with a commitment to move beyond this'. They saw as vital 'a coherent, comprehensive and cost effective framework of education beyond registration', including 'opportunities for updating knowledge and skills, bearing in mind the observation that professional knowledge is now out of date in as little as five to eight years' (Jacobi, 1976, p. 51).

Having looked at what continuing professional development is, and how it is relevant to nursing, it will be useful to consider briefly the criteria against which effective CPD can be measured. The author suggests that these should comprise:

- **the use of a range of strategies to effect learning**. If learning is to be work-related then it may be appropriate to bring it directly into the workplace, using flexible open learning delivery methods, such as that used with Health Pickup open learning packages, emanating from the NHS Training Division (NHSTD). Equally it may be appropriate to use national delivery methods such as the Royal College of Nursing (RCN) uses with *Nursing Update*, offered via BBC and the *Nursing Standard*, RCN continuing education articles in the *Nursing Standard*, *Nursing Times* Open Learning initiatives or Open University courses.
- **flexibility in terms of how, where and what the learner learns**. Learning must be needs-related in terms of both personal and professional needs (and, if we accept Madden and Mitchell's definition referred to earlier, it must also be related to the needs of employers and society) and it must fit into the learner's lifestyle. Once qualified, postregistered nurse learners are rarely full-time students. They are full-time workers, full-time family members and lead a full social life, and have to fit study around these demands.
- **acceptance of the learning that can accrue from experience**. Adults have a wealth of experience, which they bring to a learning situation, and these

experiences affect how they perceive their world. They bring a rich resource on which to base teaching and learning. Such learning is referred to as 'experiential learning'. If learners are to be encouraged to build on their prior experience, then they may need to be taught skills in reflecting critically upon it.

Kolb and Fry (1975) described an 'experiential learning cycle' (Figure 3.1), which seeks to explain how a person undergoes a concrete experience (stage 1); then looks back on the experience, reflecting on it and examining observations made at the time and subsequently (stage 2); then forms abstract concepts and generalizations as a result of the first two stages (stage 3); then tests out these ideas in new situations (stage 4). These new experimental situations then act as new concrete experiences and so the experiential learning cycle starts again.

- **reflective practice**. This is a close relative of experiential learning, which acknowledges the ways in which professionals reflect **on** action retrospectively, and also reflect **in** action as it occurs, constantly adjusting practice to 'fit' the cues that are received. Boud *et al.* (1985) suggest that reflection is a generic term that has been coined to describe 'those intellectual and affective activities in which individuals engage to explore their experiences in order to lead to new understandings and appreciations' (p. 19).

Reflective practice recognizes the knowledge that is embedded in practice (and the generation of knowledge **about** practice, not merely the application of knowledge **in** practice) – the tacit knowledge that is the domain of the intuitive expert practitioner, who often knows more than he or she can say. As Schon puts it:

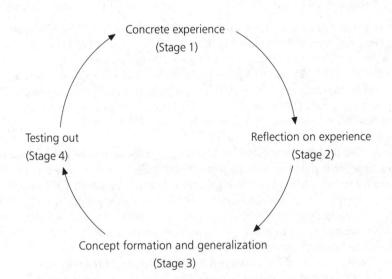

Figure 3.1 Experiential learning cycle (Kolb and Fry, 1975)

> When we go about the spontaneous, intuitive performance of the actions of everyday life, we show ourselves to be knowledgeable in a special way. Often we cannot say what it is that we know. When we try to describe it we find ourselves at a loss, or we produce descriptions that are obviously inappropriate. Our knowing is ordinarily tacit, implicit in our patterns of action and in our feel for the stuff with which we are dealing. It seems right to say that our knowing is **in** our action. (Schon, 1987, p. 49)

Benner (1984) expands on this in her discussion of expertise in nursing:

> Expertise in complex human decision making, such as nursing requires, makes the interpretation of clinical situations possible, and the knowledge embedded in this clinical expertise is central to the advancement of nursing practice and the development of nursing science. Not all the knowledge embedded in expertise can be captured in theoretical propositions. (p.30)

As Jarvis (1987) points out, if we accept this, it has profound implications for the role of the teacher who should be helping practitioners 'to crystallise the ideas they have generated in practice' (p. 50).

- **self-actualization**. The notion of meeting one's fullest potential, using education to realize personal and professional capabilities.

It should be recognized that however potentially effective the CPD itself is, success in its application depends on a 'good CPD culture', which can be seen as one of the characteristics of Handy's (1989) 'learning organization'. Cervero (1988) suggests that a culture which fosters successful CPD encompasses:

- **the existence of a positive and valuing attitude within the professional group towards lifelong learning**. It is debatable whether this exists in nursing at present. There are a number of professionally and educationally aware nurses who do value CPD, and who have the vision to see how necessary it is if we are to meet the needs of professionals, the profession, employers and society. The rest may be brought on board once CPD becomes a statutory requirement for the entire profession – and it must be borne in mind that this will not be a reality until 2001.
- **ensuring that the conditions for learning, and for responding to change are in tune with the needs of the practitioner, his or her colleagues and the organization**. One of the conditions for successful uptake of CPD opportunities is what can be referred to as 'felt need'. It is important that it is the potential consumer of CPD who perceives this need. Organizational need may well exist, but being sent to do CPD is ineffective if the learner does not see it as fitting in with his or her own needs.
- **envisaging the need for CPD, and its relevance, right from the stage of initial professional education**. The present initial preparation for nursing, as referred to earlier, will do much to help establish the need from the beginning.

- **an emphasis on helping practitioners to learn effectively**. It has to be remembered that in nursing we will be dealing with two different populations of practitioners: those who registered under the 'old' schemes of training and those who registered as a result of undertaking the present diploma level initial preparation. The latter group will have been exposed to a much wider range of educational strategies and will have been taught how to study and how to become self-directed. The former group of practitioners will not have had these advantages. It is likely that they will have experience of a fairly narrow range of teaching strategies and may have poor study techniques. The two groups will have differing needs with regard to effective learning techniques. Jarvis (1987) asserts that continuing education provision essentially should be managed by a 'highly skilled professional', and in nursing our history lends weight to this being our need.
- **The provision of support and guidance for people undertaking CPD**. This will vary between and within organizations, depending on the pervading management culture. In situations where mentorship is valued and continues beyond basic education, and where clinical supervision is seen as a key strategy for developing practice, then such support is likely. Elsewhere support may be patchy, depending on the value which managers attach to CPD. Even so, peer support can be extremely helpful.
- **seeing people (and investment in them) as an asset to the organization**. Increasing numbers of organizations are joining the government's 'Investors in People' initiative, which is used as a tool for organizational review and development. Briefly the scheme encourages employers to develop all employees so that they might more effectively achieve the objectives of the organization. While laudable on some counts, the emphasis here is on meeting organizational needs rather than those of the individual **as well as** those of the employer, and this therefore narrows the focus of CPD.

The extent to which a good culture for CPD exists within nursing is debatable. It may be salutary, therefore, to spend a little time examining how pervasive and successful CPD has become in other professions.

CONTINUING PROFESSIONAL DEVELOPMENT IN OTHER PROFESSIONS

Madden and Mitchell's study (1993) of continuing education for the professions highlights the fact that this has become a reality only since the 1980s. Prior to that time the key players, the professional bodies and institutions, were principally concerned with standard setting, controlling those who entered the profession and validating initial preparation for practice. To some extent, in a number of professions – including nursing – some of these functions have been taken over by institutions of higher education.

During the period up to the 1980s, professional development was not organized, was often spasmodic and was very much up to individual practitioners, who
relied on learned journals and organized meetings for their updating. Since the
1980s, it has come to be recognized as increasingly important, and dependent on
a partnership between professionals, their employers, the professional bodies and
higher education providers. In some cases, in particular engineering and estate
management, it has been assisted by government funding (Madden and Mitchell,
1993). Madden and Mitchell examined CPD within 20 professions grouped into
six occupational fields:

- construction
- finance and law
- engineering
- social and personal health services (including nursing)
- management
- medicine.

Their findings make interesting reading. With regard to the function of CPD:

- 95% see this as updating knowledge and skills for practice;
- 65% see this as developing new skills for practice;
- 60% see this as updating knowledge and skills outside practice;
- only 15% see it as needed for personal development and growth.

Professional bodies saw CPD as important in terms of maintaining professional
standards (25%), assessing professional competence (15%) and accrediting continuing learning (5%). Madden and Mitchell found that 70% of professional bodies
have some policy on CPD, 25% having a mandatory policy, where the sanction for
non-compliance is removal from the register, or of the right to practice, or being
reported to the relevant professional conduct committee.

- 75% of professional bodies cite the employer as funding CPD, with only 20%
  citing the individual as being responsible for meeting fees.
- 65% of professions have to meet a minimum number of hours of CPD annually, 26.8 hours being the mean.
- 35% of professional bodies set forth what is acceptable to them in relation to
  CPD undertakings.

Madden and Mitchell suggest that there are two models for CPD within the
professions: a sanctions model and a benefits model. They see the sanctions model
applying more generally to the older established professions, such as those regulated by the Law Society, the Royal Institute of British Architects, the Institute of
Chartered Accountants – and now the UKCC can be added to this list. All these
professions are setting out to demonstrate continuing professional competence,
and they see CPD as essential to maintaining up-to-date knowledge for practice,
and so sanctions will be levied against those professionals who fail to comply. The

obvious criticism of this model is that, although you can insist that someone attends a course, for example, as part of CPD, you cannot ensure that s/he learns from it or applies it to the benefit of practice.

The benefits model tends to apply in the newer or developing professions, such as social work and personnel management. Interestingly, at the time of the study the final UKCC pronouncements concerning postregistration education and practice were not yet published, and the only nursing initiative that the report authors examined was the English National Board Framework for Continuing Professional Education for Nurses, Midwives and Health Visitors (1990), which they naturally saw as a benefits model. They therefore assumed that this was the only model prevailing in nursing.

A benefits model for CPD focuses on improving professional status on a voluntary basis, together with enhancing knowledge and skills for practice outcomes, and the reward (benefit) for this is frequently a competence-based qualification (such as the ENB Higher Award). CPD is marketed to professionals in terms of advanced career opportunities. The problem with this model is that there is no guarantee that it will reach those who could most benefit from it, i.e. those who most need updating.

Continuing medical education (CME) is encouraged within a general practitioner's contract with the National Health Service by the payment of a postgraduate education allowance, established in the 1990 contracts. The allowance is paid for completion of 5 days of approved CME per year. The Royal College of General Practitioners allows that 'although these arrangements have resulted in high levels of participation, there have been doubts about the quality of educational activities and the degree of learning that has taken place' (RCGP, 1994). They go on to assert that as a Royal College they would prefer to see participation in CME recognized through a process of recertification – just as nurses are now doing.

In the past, nurse education (training) has been seen as different from that enjoyed by other professionals, and certainly as different from that of our medical colleagues. Now, however, with our move into higher education and towards becoming a graduate profession, those differences are lessening. In the realm of CPD it could be argued that we are overtaking some of the professions allied to medicine, and indeed doctors too.

In conclusion, if the aim of effective CPD is to meet the needs of a profession in maintaining and developing competence in job performance throughout the practitioners' careers, then the author would argue that CPD provision should be:

- flexible and realistic;
- based on intended learning outcomes;
- relevant to the professional needs of both practitioners and their managers;
- appropriate to differing learning styles;
- adaptable to respond to new needs quickly;
- geared to solving problems in practice, especially in relation to the client group;
- appropriate in teaching methods to adult students;

- research- or evidence-based;
- cost-effective, i.e. value for money;
- responsive to consumer evaluation;
- amenable to a variety of assessment strategies.

I shall now move from a consideration of the general to the particular and to focus on CPD within nursing, in the context of the professional changes that have taken place in the last decade.

CONTINUING PROFESSIONAL DEVELOPMENT WITHIN NURSING

Having been introduced generally to CPD, the focus now narrows somewhat, to examine what was going on in relation to CPD in nursing in the first half of this present decade – and here the term 'nursing' is used in the specific sense, rather than the generic, for it is not proposed to examine the situation within midwifery.

At the time of writing, continuing professional development is very much a reality in nursing – everybody knows that it is part of what they have to do, if not now, then by 2001. How did we reach this point?

The coming of postregistration education and practice (PREP)

In October 1990 the UKCC published *The Report of the Post-registration Education and Practice Project*, which came to be known as the PREPP report. The project group, in August 1989, had been set the task of 'developing a coherent and comprehensive framework for education and practice beyond registration' (UKCC, 1990, p. 10). The result, following a discussion paper in January 1990, was a consultative document that was commented on widely in the professional press and was also responded to by the profession, both by individuals and by organizations.

After much discussion and some wrangling between professional organizations, the UKCC and the Department of Health, three and a half years later, in March 1994, the PREPP proposals culminated in the publication by the UKCC of *The Future of Professional Practice – the Council's Standards for Education and Practice Following Registration*. This time gap was much longer than anticipated by the profession, and it was to be extended by a further year before the contents of the report became law and began to be enacted on 1 April 1995.

In every edition of the UKCC's Code of Professional Conduct, from the time the UKCC was set up, there was a clause that required practitioners to 'maintain and improve your professional knowledge and competence'. The 1992 edition (UKCC, 1992b), however, was quite unequivocal about this, stating that this **must** be done, whereas in the 1984 edition it stated that practitioners 'shall take every reasonable opportunity' to do so – arguably a less demanding statement. The main focus of PREPP was on this maintenance and improvement of knowledge and competence.

The 1990 proposals

The PREPP report set the proposed changes within the context of professional practice, examining demographic trends, epidemiological changes, lifestyle and health inequalities and the NHS and Community Care Act of the same year. This latter was to set in motion the most radical overhaul that the NHS had seen since its inception, alongside accompanying changes in the ways in which nurse education was to be delivered within the internal markets that were developing. The project team recommended five main proposals.

- Between 3 and 6 months' support should be supplied for the newly registered practitioner, in order to consolidate the learning outcomes achieved at registration, by a preceptor who has been prepared for the role.
- All practitioners must be able to demonstrate that they have maintained and developed their professional knowledge and competence. They should record this development in a personal professional profile. The team suggested that every practitioner should have opportunities to learn, which should be part of a credit accumulation and transfer system. Each practitioner should have a minimum of 5 days' study leave every 3 years (this wording was to change subtly in future versions of PREPP), in order to be eligible for periodic reregistration. The project team stated that this updating should be verified by 'a named, experienced practitioner', who would provide a signed statement to the Council to this effect.
- After a break in practice of 5 years or more practitioners were to complete a return to practice programme approved by a National Board.
- After registration the team saw practice as a continuum, divided into:

  - primary – the period following preceptor support;
  - advanced – involving direct care, education, research, management, health policy-making, leadership and strategy development;
  - consultant – pioneer roles as authoritative resources and innovators.

Earlier in this chapter mention was made of the publication in 1986 of the UKCC's plans for a new initial preparation for practice, commonly known then as Project 2000. It was clear that if education in preparation for practice was to be set at diploma level, then education following registration had to be set at a higher level – first-degree and potentially beyond. This was an issue that UKCC failed to address specifically within the initial PREPP proposals, simply stating that the Council 'will from time to time agree the standard, kind and content of preparation to meet the demands of practice' (p. 27). In relation to the consultant role the group stated that 'there can be no prescribed pattern of education and experience' (p. 28). This section of the PREPP proposals was to change significantly by the final version.

- To be eligible to practice practitioners must, in addition to the foregoing requirements relating to updating and returning to practice after a break:

– pay their periodic fee;
– submit a notification to practice.

Response to the 1990 PREPP proposals

One of the key questions that was being asked following the release of the report was 'Who pays?' In response to this, Price Waterhouse were commissioned by UKCC to study and analyse the costs and benefits of PREPP, so that the government could be given precise figures in order to decide whether to fund the proposals. A UKCC press statement (UKCC, 1991) stated that the proposals would cost between £50m and £100m per year, and Carlisle (1991) suggested that 800 000 working days would be lost to study leave.

Trevor Clay, late General Secretary of the Royal College of Nursing, expressed the concern that many were feeling:

> For 50 years nurses have been fighting for reform throughout all spheres of nurse education. I feel Project 2000 should be clearly debated and settled before the advance towards PREPP is implemented ... . The ultimate responsibility will eventually fall upon the shoulders of the individual nurse, which is yet another erosion of any salary increases they may receive.

Tom Bolger, then Director of Education at the Royal College of Nursing, broadly welcomed the proposals, but questioned the three tiers of nurses that the report proposed (Meehan, 1990).

Practitioners were reported to feel angry about the possibility of finding themselves responsible for paying for their own continuing professional development, but a note of resignation regarding this was beginning to creep in (Sims, 1991).

Generally the focus on the part of practitioners seemed to be on the required 5 study days, rather than on the other four recommendations. There was concern – and there still is – that the stipulated minimum might become the maximum (Carlisle, 1991), although Professor Margaret Green, who chaired the project, insisted that it was nurses themselves who were adamant that a figure be included to quantify professional updating (Friend, 1991), so that those who then had no CPD had something to aim for. Practitioners were also voicing concern about the staffing levels necessary to support newly registered nurses, and the need for effective monitoring; about who would verify the personal professional profiles; about 5 days of updating being too short a period of 'time allowed' (nurses still seemed to think that they might be given time for CPD); and about return to practice programmes being necessary after a 3-year break in service rather than 5 years (McHale, 1992).

In May 1992 the UKCC published its proposals for the future of community education and practice (UKCC, 1992c). It set out to offer a means of reshaping education for nurses within community health care. During educational preparation for community health-care practice it recommended core shared modules where appropriate, followed by modules geared to individual role preparation to meet specific needs in specific situations. The essence of this was later to appear in the UKCC's final statements on PREPP in 1994. In financial terms this was less contentious, since it was not suggested that nurses working in the community fund these proposed educational shifts themselves.

In July 1992 the Health Minister, Baroness Cumberlege, personally attended the UKCC meeting to apologize for the government's delay in offering financial support for PREPP, while reaffirming its unreserved support for the underlying principles. In a letter to the UKCC she suggested that the government would need to come up with a system for costing PREPP by the end of 1992 (Castledine, 1992). By 1993, however, a decision with regard to funding the professional updating aspects of PREPP was still awaited from the government. Colin Ralph, then Registrar of the UKCC, asserted that the outlay would only be 'modest'. He was quoted (Allen, 1993) as describing PREPP as 'an important investment in practitioners at the centre of patient care' and expressed confidence that, after debate, ministers would agree to foot the bill.

At this point there began to be less emphasis on 'study days' and more talk from the UKCC about 'a day spent in a professional library' constituting study activity (UKCC, 1993) – a subtle move away from provision for nurses by employers. The UKCC, determined not to be too prescriptive about what might be deemed as suitable activities for updating, suggested five categories of relevance, with a range of activities and study content relevant to each:

- **reducing risk**: health promotion identification, protection of individuals, risk reduction, health promotion, screening, heightening of awareness;
- **care enhancement**: developments in clinical practice and treatments, new techniques and approaches to care, standard setting, empowering consumers;
- **patient, client and colleague support** (note that by 1994 this was to include also 'family', and by 1995 'family' had inexplicably disappeared): counselling services, leadership for professional practice, supervision of clinical practice;
- **practice development**: external visits, exchange arrangements, personal research/study, briefing on health and professional policy change, service audit;
- **education development**: external visits, exchange arrangements, personal study/research, educational audit, teaching and learning skills.

Without explanation it can be seen that such a list is of little help to the majority of practitioners, and at its worst it is confusing. For example, in what respect are 'counselling services' part of professional updating? Is it assumed that the practitioner is learning about them? Offering them? Consuming them? And what of 'supervision of clinical practice'? One assumes that the UKCC is suggesting that the practitioner undergoes supervision, as part of his/her continuing professional development – or does it mean s/he offers supervision? At the time of writing, some practitioners are using these categories as portfolio section headings; others see little use for them.

In truth, many of the communications that emanated from the UKCC in relation to PREPP were not user-friendly. They lacked a direct, clear, informative style, which would have enabled practitioners to see from the start how they could best use opportunities for continuing professional development. It was not until March 1995, in *PREP and YOU*, that practitioners received full and clear instructions, just before the requirements were due to start for some practitioners.

The Future of Professional Practice – the Council's Standards for Education and Practice following Registration

In March 1994 the UKCC published this final report – the culmination of widespread consultation with the profession and the resulting amendments – which brought together the initial generic PREPP proposals and those later ones relating to nurses working in community health care. Here, for the first time, the UKCC acknowledges that this continuing provision is based on the initial diploma-level preparation for practice. With this has to come the acceptance that later tiers of education must be at first-degree level and beyond.

Interestingly, the parts of the report that stirred up the greatest debate within the press and most of the profession are contained in just five of the 49 pages. Those five pages relate to maintaining effective registration with the Council and cover:

- **undertaking 'a minimum of 5 days (or equivalent) study for professional development every 3 years'**, stating that this can be as whole days or part-time equivalents, not usually undertaken as a course, but spread over time as relevant to the individual practitioner's needs and work. The Council suggests that, whether the study is formal or not, objectives are set, and for formal study (such as attending a conference) the participant pays attention to the relevance of the content, the credibility of the teachers/speakers and the objectives and evaluation of the initiative.
- **notification of practice** in order for the Council to be able to record a practitioner's qualifications and area of practice.
- **return to practice programmes** approved by the national Boards when there has been a break in practice of in the region of 5 years.
- **keeping a personal professional profile** 'to help practitioners to identify their personal and practice-related study needs and then to choose the relevant activity to meet such needs.' Details given at this stage regarding the profile were sparse and no reference was made to earlier suggestions that the UKCC would itself be supplying profiles to the profession. In 1993 Maggy Wallace, then Assistant Registrar at the UKCC, was saying 'practitioners will complete a personal professional profile, the basis of which will be issued by the UKCC as part of the UKCC personal file' (Wallace, 1993). This would clearly have been an expensive undertaking that, by 1994, the UKCC was not prepared to fund. The earlier proposal that the profile be countersigned and verified by a professional who would be accountable to UKCC had similarly disappeared. By this stage it had been accepted that self-verification with audit would be professionally more acceptable – and feasible.

The remainder of the 1994 report focuses (briefly) on preceptorship and (lengthily) on specialist and advanced practice in relation to nursing, midwifery and community health care, together with standards for education, teaching and transitional arrangements, with particular reference to a range of specialist areas. It suggests that preparation for specialist practice be set at first-degree level, and at master's level for advanced practice.

The response of the profession in 1994

The weekly nursing journals published summaries and possible timetables for implementation on their news pages at the time the report was published during the week of 2 March, but there was nothing in the way of substantive analyses. It was as if all the talking had been done and the profession now accepted the changes, and even the fact that no money appeared to be forthcoming from the Department of Health to support implementation, due – subject to legislation – on 1 April 1995.

During 1994 the UKCC issued, in *Register* (their information bulletin sent to all registered practitioners), a proposed timetable for implementation of PREPP and indicated that a series of information sheets (which in fact never materialized) would be available from early 1995. They promised fact sheets (which did materialize) in Spring 1995.

From the personal experience of the author it was quite clear that in the latter part of 1994 and during spring 1995 there was immense uncertainty and anxiety on the part of many nurses about what PREPP meant for them in practical terms. Many were labouring under the delusion that, for example, all nurses would need to start meeting the requirements for professional updating from 1 April 1995, whereas this would not begin to apply to all practitioners until 1 April 2001. Some thought that they would have to attend (and pay for) five actual study days or conferences. Others thought that mere certificates of attendance would be enough to satisfy the UKCC. Many saw the profile as a glorified *curriculum vitae*. Yet others were unsure how to start the profiling process.

March 1995: the final guidelines – a critique

In late March 1995 the UKCC sent to every registered practitioner, both in the UK and abroad, a series of eight fact sheets entitled *PREP and YOU: Maintaining Your Registration Standards for Education Following Registration*. Interestingly, the words 'and practice' have been deleted in this version, after 'education', on the cover sheet. Whether this is simply an omission is not clear.

A question and answer format is used throughout to cover the content. Certainly there is an attempt to use clear, direct speech and to explain why some of the requirements are pertinent – for example, under 'Why do you need to complete a Notification of Practice form?' follows the explanation that this will help UKCC to 'identify the number and type of qualifications being used in practice; the number of people in specific areas of practice; and the number of people practising in specific employment sectors, for example, in mental health nursing.' In these fact sheets, more than anywhere else before, the UKCC tries to help practitioners to understand what PREPP is really about.

Throughout, the ball is put clearly in the individual practitioner's court: 'You are responsible for seeking opportunities to learn and to improve the level of your competence in the interests of patient and client care' (Fact Sheet 3). There is a potentially useful section that sets out to help practitioners plan their professional development, suggesting stages such as:

1. Review your competence … and identify where you want to develop.
2. Set your learning objectives … what do you want to achieve to help you to develop?
3. Develop an action plan … select your learning activities.
4. Implement your action plan … involve your manager or supervisor, negotiate study time and, if necessary, help with funding. (There is later an expanded section on negotiating study leave and funding.)
5. Evaluation … How good was the initiative which you undertook? Did you meet your objectives? Was what you learned of use in practice? How can you share what you have learned?
6. Record your study time and learning outcomes.

Fact Sheet 4 focuses on 'Your personal professional profile' and contains the first recorded account, in detail, of how the UKCC sees this. The Council perceives the profile as having two functions:

• helping the practitioner to identify and value his/her strengths and achievements;
• acting as a source of information for the UKCC and the practitioner about CPD.

It states that the profile is different from a CV and from a portfolio; it differentiates it from the latter by suggesting that a portfolio 'normally contains evidence of educational and professional achievement such as project work and published articles and papers'. I have some difficulty with this, since it seems to be saying that educational and professional achievements (such as project work and published articles and papers) would not, therefore, be suitable for inclusion as evidence of professional updating, as they are part of a portfolio, rather than a profile. But why should an article not be suitable evidence? It would seem to be the culmination of personal research and study, which are suggested, in Fact Sheet 3, for inclusion in the categories of both Practice Development and Education Development.

The UKCC goes on to say that the profile is a personal document and that much of what it contains is private and confidential. Given this and also that the UKCC has a statutory right to ensure that practitioners are abiding by the requirements for professional updating, the statement on p. 4 of Fact Sheet 4 is somewhat odd: that the UKCC may request information on 'your strengths and weaknesses'. It is not a statutory duty of UKCC to record practitioners' strengths and weaknesses. It would, in fact, seem that UKCC are using the terms 'portfolio' and 'profile' in a confused and confusing way. Brown (1992) offers a definition for each that is straightforward and commonly accepted: a personal portfolio is:

> a private collection of evidence which demonstrates the continuing acquisition of skills, knowledge, attitudes, understanding and achievement. It is both retrospective and prospective, as well as reflecting the current stage of development and activity of the individual. (p. 1–2)

Whereas a profile is:

> a collection of evidence which is selected from the personal portfolio for a particular purpose and a particular audience. (p. 4)

The UKCC is, therefore, more correctly asking practitioners to keep a personal and private portfolio, from which they will extract a personal professional profile for the purposes of assuring UKCC that they have met the PREPP requirements.

SHOULD CONTINUING PROFESSIONAL DEVELOPMENT BE MANDATORY OR VOLUNTARY? THE AMERICAN EXPERIENCE

This may seem a redundant question in view of the decision by the UKCC, discussed earlier in this chapter, to opt for a mandatory model for CPD for nurses, midwives and health visitors in the UK. However, the issues still bear examination in the light of considerable experience with mandatory continuing education (CE) for nurses in some of the states of the USA.

In 1991 Casey undertook a study visit to USA to investigate mandatory continuing education, which had been in place in a number of states, for nurses, since the 1970s (Casey, 1991). This initiative, within the USA, has to be seen within the context of an established system of continuing education for millions of workers.

In 1968 a National Task Force was set up in North America to examine the feasibility of developing a national unit of educational currency to measure continuing education. It designated the continuing education unit (CEU) for this purpose. The CEU 'represents ten contact hours of participation in an organized continuing education experience under responsible sponsorship, capable direction and qualified instruction' (Council on the Continuing Education Unit – now the International Association for Continuing Education and Training – definition, used on current publicity leaflets from IACET).

In some states of the USA there are mandatory requirements not only about hours of study but also about topics studied – for example, in some states sessions on AIDS or child abuse are compulsory (Casey, 1991).

Continuing education for nurses in the USA was at different stages of development in virtually every state in the early 1970s. The ANA, therefore, via its

Commission on Nursing Education, took steps to standardize this situation. Its guidelines were approved in 1975 by the Council on Continuing Education and the CEU was adopted as the nursing currency.

Although the majority of states (all but two) accept ANA-approved CE initiatives, each state board continues to offer its own interpretation of CE with which nurses in that state have to comply.

The American Nurses Association was among the first of the organizations in the USA to adopt the CEU and to endorse mandatory CE for nurses. Today, contact hours rather than CEUs are used (ANCC, 1994), and since 1985 the ANA has embraced the view that individual practitioners are responsible for identifying their own needs for CE and accountable for meeting these needs (Carpenito, 1991a).

Just under half of the states require mandatory CE, annual requirements ranging from $7\frac{1}{2}$ hours to 15 contact hours (with 50 minutes representing one contact hour; Casey, 1991). It should be noted that the requirements of the UKCC are broadly in line with American thinking (i.e. about 30 hours – 5 days – of study over 3 years).

The American Nurses Association believes (*inter alia*) that:

(a) professional development needs are influenced by the nurse's acceptance of accountability and responsibility for his or her own practice;
(b) lifelong learning is essential for nurses to maintain and increase competence in nursing practice;
(c) many educational options are necessary to meet the diverse needs of the nursing population;
(d) that nursing continuing education and staff development, based on adult learning principles, contribute to professional development. (ANA, 1994, pp. 2–3).

These beliefs echo what has been said by other writers, and the UKCC, earlier in this dissertation, and they underpin the UKCC's guidelines in *The Future of Professional Practice* (UKCC, 1994).

The ANA sets six standards against which it can measure effective provision of CE offerings, together with criteria for the achievement of each:

- **Standard 1**: Administration of the provider unit is consistent with the organization's mission, philosophy, purpose and goals. The organizational structure facilitates the provision of learning activities for nurses.
- **Standard 2**: Qualified administrative, educational and support personnel are responsible for achieving the goals of the provider unit.
- **Standard 3**: Material resources and facilities are adequate to achieve the goals and implement the functions of the provider unit.
- **Standard 4**: Principles of education and adult learning are used to design educational activities.
- **Standard 5**: The provider unit establishes and maintains a record-keeping and report system.
- **Standard 6**: The professional development educator role is practised in a man-

ner that enhances learners' competence to provide quality health care and their contributions to the profession (ANA, 1994).

In 1989 the ANA set up a subsidiary called the American Nurses' Credentialing Center (ANCC), which handles both accreditation and approval of CE initiatives for nurses, based on the foregoing standards.

In the light of an examination of the ANA standards relating to CE in the USA, and a consideration of their potential usefulness, the question remains as to why the UKCC did not adopt a similar approach here. This is especially pertinent since *The Future of Professional Practice – The Council's Standards for Education and Practice following Registration* (UKCC, 1994) set standards for specialist practice and education but not for professional updating activities. Clearly, practitioners would have been assured of a basic level of provision from all providers of CPD had the UKCC chosen this route.

However, there have always been differences of opinion in the USA with regard to whether or not CE should actually be mandatory, and whether it has tangible benefits in practice (Casey, 1991). As del Bueno (1976, p. 136) suggested:

[E]ducation, either basic or continuing, should not be used as a panacea for either the problems of nursing practice or health care delivery. Used judiciously for the proper problems, education can be an appropriate treatment. Used inappropriately education can only be a costly failure.

This quotation should be borne in mind when considering Puetz's (1983) study of the uptake of CE in Indiana. Puetz attempted to replicate an earlier (1975) study, looking at which nurses actually took up CE offerings. She found that those who undertook CE opportunities were younger, better educated, worked in acute settings and were of higher professional status than those who chose not to undertake CE. This fits with Madden and Mitchell's (1993) suggestion that those who most need CPD, with a voluntary, benefits model, are not necessarily those who access it. Puetz's research convinced the Indiana authorities that mandatory CE in nursing was needed; however, the legislation had to be dropped as a result of nurses' protests.

As Casey suggests, it was envisaged in the USA that by the 1980s all states would implement mandatory CE. This did not, however, come to pass, and in some instances, notably Colorado, mandatory CE for nurses has been repealed after 12 years (National Council of State Boards of Nursing, 1994), although this was reported to be met with mixed feelings – lack of widespread opportunities and expense were cited by those opposed to the concept, while those with whom the notion found favour saw public protection as a key reason for a mandatory approach. Interestingly, the Colorado State Board is putting the saved resources to use in developing nurses 'who practice in a substandard manner' (p. 5), while acknowledging that every nurse is accountable for his/her level of competence.

After 12 years, the findings in Colorado were that nurses, in fact, did much more CE than they were charged to do; no nurse had ever been identified as unsafe throughout the CE programme; 100% compliance was achieved (bar one nurse);

nurses seemed more concerned about whether a CE initiative was approved than about whether it would improve practice; but the number of disciplinary actions for substandard care continued to escalate. These actions are reported to be concerned with problems in the delivery of basic nursing functions such as documentation, giving medications and poor handwashing, rather than with the use of new technology. There did not seem to be, therefore, a compelling reason to continue with a compulsory approach.

In 1991, when mandatory continuing education was first mooted as a possibility in the UK, following the UKCC's initial PREPP discussion papers, Carpenito put forward the case for why coercion does not work, either in terms of improving practice or in terms of benefits to nurses themselves. She did say, however, that a tangible result in the USA has been the improvement and increase in provision of CE opportunities (Carpenito, 1991a). However, as she asserts, for those who are not self-directed and motivated to learn, making CE mandatory will not make such practitioners learn, even though it may make them go through the motions of attending CE initiatives.

What will ensure competence to practise is not mandatory CE but a commitment to lifelong learning (Carpenito, 1991b). Carpenito sees mandatory CE as at odds with the values and beliefs on which lifelong learning is based. She argues that frequently it can be aimed at the 'lowest common denominator' of practitioners rather than being targeted at the needs of those who are already competent in basic concepts and who have identified more advanced learning needs based on process rather than content – for example, problem-solving or decision-making – rather than learning focused on task mastery.

CONCLUSION

At the start of this chapter reference was made to the UKCC's consistent requirement that nurses maintain their professional knowledge and competence. Continuing professional development activities that attempt to enhance knowledge would not seem to be in short supply. A cursory glance through the listings and advertisements in the professional press would assure one of this. What, though, of CPD initiatives that attempt to enhance competence in the workplace? These would seem to be less plentiful. It would be a pity if we failed to capitalize on the opportunity we have to benefit and develop nursing practice, through the move to CPD and lifelong learning initiated by the UKCC's PREPP requirements. PREPP will almost certainly result in personal and professional development for those who undertake its mandatory requirements, through portfolio development; practice, too, should derive benefit through more CPD opportunities designed specifically to extend its boundaries.

REFERENCES

Allen, D. (1993) The Cost of PREP. *Nursing Standard*, **7**(23), 5.

ANA (1994) *Standards for Nursing Professional Development: Continuing Education and Staff Development*, American Nurses Association, Washington, DC.

ANCC (1994) *Accreditation of Continuing Education in Nursing*, American Nurses Credentialing Center, Washington, DC.

Benner, P. (1984) *From Novice to Expert*, Addison-Wesley, Menlo Park, CA.

Boud, D., Keogh, R. and Walker, D. (1985) *Reflection: Turning Experience into Learning*, Kogan Page, London.

Brookfield, S. (1986) *Understanding and Facilitating Adult Learning: A Comprehensive Analysis of Principles and Effective Practices*, Open University Press, Milton Keynes.

Brown, R. (1992) *Portfolio Development and Profiling for Nurses*, Quay Publishing, Lancaster.

Carlisle, D. (1991) Take five. *Nursing Times*, **87**(6), 40–41.

Carpenito, J. (1991a) Why coercion does not work. *Nursing Times*, **87**(47), 29–31.

Carpenito, J. (1991b) A lifetime of commitment. *Nursing Times*, **87**(48), 53–55.

Casey, N. (1991) Report of a study visit to investigate continuing education in the United States of America, unpublished.

Castledine, G. (1992) PREP: gaining momentum or slowing down? *British Journal of Nursing*, **1**(8), 371.

Cervero, R. (1988) *Effective Continuing Education for Professionals*, Jossey-Bass, San Francisco, CA.

Council on the Continuing Education Unit (1979) *Criteria and Guidelines for Use of the Continuing Education Unit*, Council on the Continuing Education Unit, Washington, DC, cited in Casey (1991).

Cropley, A. (1981) Lifelong learning: a rationale for teacher training. *Journal of Education for Teaching*, **7**.

Davies, C. (1995) *Gender and the Professional Predicament in Nursing*, Open University Press, Buckingham.

Del Bueno, D. (1976) The effect of continuing education on on-the-job behaviour in Continuing Education in Nursing – a prospectus, in *Proceedings of the National Conference, Kansas, American Nurses Association*, November, pp. 133–141.

English National Board for Nursing, Midwifery and Health Visiting (1990) *Framework for Continuing Professional Education*, London, ENB.

Friend, B. (1991) View from the top. *Nursing Times*, **87**(8), 24–25.

Handy, C. (1989) *The Age of Unreason*, Century Business, London.

Hinchliff, S. (1994) Learning for life. *Nursing Standard*, **48**(8), 20–21.

Houle, C. (1980) *Continuing Learning in the Professions*, Jossey-Bass, San Francisco, CA.

Hunt, E. (ed.) (1992) *Professional Workers as Learners*, US Department of Education, Washington, DC.

Jacobi, E. (1976) *The Status of Continuing Education Programmes for Nurses in the United States*, King Edward's Hospital Fund, London, cited in UKCC, 1986.

Jarvis, P. (1984) Continuing education. *Journal of District Nursing*, **3**(12), 14–16.

Jarvis, P. (1987) Lifelong education and its relevance to nursing. *Nurse Education Today*, **7**, 49–55.

Jolley, M. (1989) The professionalisation of nursing: the uncertain path, in *Current Issues in Nursing*, (eds M. Jolley and P. Allen), Chapman & Hall, London.

Knapper, C. and Cropley, A. (1991) *Lifelong Learning and Higher Education*, 2nd edn, Routledge, London.

Knowles, M. (1984) *The Adult Learner: A Neglected Species*, 3rd edn, Gulf Publishing, Houston, TX.

Kolb, D. and Fry, R. (1975) Towards an applied theory of experiential learning, in *Theories of Group Processes*, (ed. C. Cooper), John Wiley & Sons, Chichester.

Lorentzon, M. (1991) *Professionalism and Professionalisation*, Distance Learning Centre, South Bank University, London.

Madden, C. and Mitchell, V. (1993) *Professions, Standards and Competence: A Survey of Continuing Education for the Professions*, University of Bristol Department for Continuing Education, Bristol.

McHale, C. (1992) Nurses' responses to PREP: a short study. *Nursing Standard*, **6**(31), 33–36.

Meehan, F. (1990) PREPP: a future framework. *Nursing*, **4**(23), 5–6.

National Council of State Boards of Nursing (1994) Mandatory Continuing Education for Nurses Repealed in Colorado. *Newsletter of the National Council*, **15**(2), 5–6.

Puetz, P. (1983) Legislating a continuing education requirement for licensure renewal. *Journal of Continuing Education in Nursing*, **14**(5), 5–12.

RCGP (1994) *Education and Training for General Practice*, Royal College of General Practitioners, London.

Schon, D. (1983) *The Reflective Practitioner*, Basic Books, New York.

Sims, J. (1991) From the sharp end. *Nursing Times*, **87**(8), 26–28.

UKCC (1986) *Project 2000: A New Preparation for Practice*, United Kingdom Central Council for Nursing, Midwifery and Health Visiting, London.

UKCC (1990) *The Report of the Post-registration Education and Practice Project*, United Kingdom Central Council for Nursing, Midwifery and Health Visiting, London.

UKCC (1991) *Post registration and Practice – The Next Steps* (press statement), United Kingdom Central Council for Nursing, Midwifery and Health Visiting, London.

UKCC (1992b) *Code of Professional Conduct*, 3rd edn, United Kingdom Central Council for Nursing, Midwifery and Health Visiting, London.

UKCC (1992a) *The Scope of Professional Practice*, United Kingdom Central Council for Nursing, Midwifery and Health Visiting, London.

UKCC (1992c) *Report on Proposals for the Future of Community Education and Practice*, United Kingdom Central Council for Nursing, Midwifery and Health Visiting, London.

UKCC (1993) *Final Proposals for the Future of Post-registration Education and Practice*, United Kingdom Central Council for Nursing, Midwifery and Health Visiting, London.

UKCC (1994) *The Future of Professional Practice: The Council's Standards for Education and Practice following Registration*, United Kingdom Central Council for Nursing, Midwifery and Health Visiting, London.

UKCC (1995) *PREP and YOU: Maintaining Your Registration Standards for Education Following Registration*, United Kingdom Central Council for Nursing, Midwifery and Health Visiting, London.

Wallace, M. (1993) Preparing for the future. *Nursing Times*, **89**(31), 42–44.

The wider context of continuing education

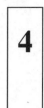

Stella Parker

CONTINUING EDUCATION IN HIGHER EDUCATION

Most professions now accept that two or three years of full-time initial higher education and training is not sufficient to last a lifetime. Professional knowledge and skills are constantly changing, professional competencies are continually increasing, and in some cases the core operational functions of a profession have changed radically over the past decade or so. Supporters of lifelong learning argue that the ability to cope with these occupational changes is enhanced if people have the opportunities to continue with education and training throughout their working lives. In the early 1980s many professions in the UK gradually began to encourage their members to engage in continuing professional development (CPD) and since then this gradual approach has become accelerated (Madden and Mitchell, 1993). Watts's survey (1996) makes this point; she surveyed 20 occupational groups who control entry to their group and (in most cases) control their right to practice. Using these two criteria as an (admittedly) crude indicator of a profession, her results show that 15 of these professions either require or strongly recommend that their members take up CPD programmes and, of the remaining five, two are evaluating their CPD requirements with a view to intensifying them. The nursing profession is included in the first 15 along with architects, solicitors and surveyors.

The professions are not alone in their appetite for postinitial education and training – many other occupational groups and adults in general have greatly increased their participation all forms of postcompulsory education and training over the last two decades. This is an international phenomenon that has occurred in many other industrialized countries (Hore, 1993) and the reasons are as yet imperfectly understood. The general term now used in the UK to encompass the educational and training provision for adults is continuing education. Continuing education is generally described as any formal education or training that is taken up after an interval following the end of continuous initial education. Continuing education thus covers a wide range of adult educational opportunities that can take place in numerous locations, including private providers as well as institutions of further and/or higher education and colleges of adult education. Within the UK's system of higher education, continuing education covers:

- full-time and part-time undergraduate degree and diploma courses;
- vocational or professional courses that can lead to qualifications;
- non-award-bearing, liberal adult education courses;
- courses designed to facilitate entry into higher education, generally known as access courses (Davies, 1995).

Davies's list (above) represents a wide spectrum of activities, not all of which are exclusively for returning adults, and indeed adults participating in the first two often find themselves sitting alongside younger, traditional students who have gone straight on from school to higher education. Davies's list of programmes can be defined as either continuing education or traditional provision depending on whether or not adult returning students are enrolled on them. This is the crux of a dilemma when trying to define continuing education in higher education because the definition appears to depend on whether or not the students are defined as adults. One way out of this dilemma is to distinguish between full-time provision and part-time provision; continuing education is usually part-time provision in higher education.

There is now a reasonable body of knowledge about many aspects of adult participation in part-time education and training. For example, we know which groups of adults are likely to participate in formal learning activities, their reasons for participation, when and where much of their learning takes place. Adult learners often choose what to learn and, if the formal system does not suit their needs, they will engage in non-formal, self-directed learning episodes, and there is some evidence from research that provides an understanding of these activities too. The diversity of this knowledge about adults as learners – i.e. the why, when, where and what – forms the basis of the recognized academic field of continuing education. It is a field rather than a discipline, because it draws upon other disciplines (which include psychology, history, social science, philosophy and, to some extent, economics and policy studies) and applies them to the study of the education of adults.

It is possible to engage in this academic field of continuing education both as a practising teacher and as a researcher. For practising teachers, there are training courses that draw upon the knowledge of good practice in the design and delivery of continuing education programmes, but there are problems with theorizing about the processes of adult learning. There is no single theory that explains how adults learn, but there is a repertoire of knowledge about factors that influence their learning. In spite of the fact that practitioners know they are doing something different when they teach adults there is no solid body of theory to underpin this practice. The best that practitioners can do is to be knowledgeable about the many theoretical perspectives (some of which appear contradictory) relating to the education of adults and to use them as a basis to inform practice, in the light of contextual circumstances.

Continuing education in higher education is inevitably influenced by factors similar to those that influence and control other fields and disciplines in universities. According to Clark's (1983) transnational analysis there are three main factors that influence the form and functions of higher education – the State, the market and the academic oligarchy. These three are used in this chapter as a basis for examining developments and trends in continuing education, but their meanings here are interpreted rather narrowly. The State is interpreted as the government and a set of publicly financed institutions, the latter not necessarily working in harmony with the government but working to its agenda (Dale, 1989). The market for continuing education is here interpreted as those who undertake and generally pay for all or some of their programmes of continuing education – in other words, the adult learners. Employers influence the market too, but in the UK only about 10% of vocational higher continuing education is delivered by universities, and within this employers have a limited role (Maguire *et al.*, 1993). Finally, the academic oligarchy refers collectively to the agents who control the continuing education curriculum, and for professional courses there are two agents discussed in this chapter – the university academics and the practitioners representing the professional organizations.

THE INFLUENCE OF THE STATE

Occupational relevance and equality of opportunity

The idea that a highly educated and trained workforce can deliver a successful national economy is not a new one, and the criticisms of British schools, colleges and universities for failing to deliver work-related education are not new either. As far back as 1690 an anonymous writer reflected on the poor quality of goods produced by English artisans and concluded that their failings were due to the limited initial education and subsequent sparse vocational training of the workforce when compared to other countries (Aldcroft, 1992). This anonymous writer was living before the establishment of the British State education system, so direct comparisons cannot be made between then and now, but nonetheless similar criticisms have been levelled at the system ever since its inception. In 1868 the first major report on schooling (the Taunton Report) recommended that useful subjects should be included in the curriculum and that less time should be spent on classical subjects. Over the next 70 years or so there were many other reports, e.g. the Samuelson

Report (1882–1884), the Bryce Commission (1895) and the Hadow Report (1926), all of which echoed the case for education to be vocationally relevant and also for expanding equal opportunities by making secondary education universal. By the beginning of the Second World War, all British children were required to attend secondary school but the majority left at the age of 14 years. Unless they then entered an apprenticeship they had very few possibilities of any further training or education provided by their employers. There were possibilities for part-time study in their own time, and in the 1930s over 2 million youngsters enrolled each year for night classes that were directly relevant to their employment.

The educational policies of all British governments since 1945 have been underpinned by these two themes identified in the aforementioned reports – firstly, the commitment to equality of opportunity and secondly, the need to remedy the perceived failure of the British educational system at all levels to be vocationally relevant (Burrage, 1994). The first theme, focusing as it did on access to secondary education in the first decades of this century, shifted in later years to accessing tertiary education (Halsey, 1993). The second theme (vocational education and training) was reiterated in the Crowther Report of 1959, which recommended the establishment of a national training structure, but this was not put into place. In the 1960s, the State's attention and resources were consumed with the expansion of the (then) academically oriented tertiary sector of education, while strategies for developing vocational education and training remained a peripheral issue.

For adults in general and for the professions too, one consequence of raising initial educational attainment levels is that demands for more advanced studies generally follow, and the brief description below illustrates this point by examining recent national trends in access and occupational relevance in higher education.

Equality of opportunity – adult access to higher education since 1945

Government measures to increase adult access to higher education were put into place immediately after the Second World War when 60 000 extra university places were made available to those returning from the armed services (Benn and Fieldhouse, 1993). In 1963, the Robbins Report recommended an expansion of the higher education system and this led immediately to the establishment of nine new universities and the elevation of ten Colleges of Advanced Technology to university status. By the end of the 1960s, 31 polytechnics and 14 Central Scottish Institutes had become designated as higher education institutions and the Open University (OU) had emerged. The OU was designated specifically as a university for part-time adult students and today enrols over 200 000 students per annum (HEFCE, 1996a).

The developments that originated in the Robbins Report were unprecedented in the history of British higher education – as well as increasing participation rates (mostly for younger students), universities and polytechnics were given parity of esteem. For continuing education the relevance of Robbins is that the State provided an expanded infrastructure, and once this was in place part-time adult students began to take advantage of it. Consequently over the past 20 years an even more rapid period of growth in adult participation has occurred, but this time it was led not by the State but by the market. Student enrolments in general have doubled since 1975 (Smithers and Robinson, 1995) so that currently there are almost 1.5 million students (HEFCE, 1996b). This increase is due firstly to a growth in participation rates of returning adults who, by the late 1980s, began to outnumber the younger entrants to higher education for the first time (Parry, 1995). The second factor is the participation of 18/19-year-olds, 30% or more of whom now progress from school to higher education (Smithers and Robinson, 1995).

The most recent figures available indicate that the trend shown by returning adults is continuing and now increasing numbers of adults are enrolling as post-experience or postgraduate part-time students. Adult students are now in the majority on non-degree courses (certificates, diplomas and non-accredited courses) and altogether they represent 28% of total university enrolments (HEFCE, 1996b). The demands made by adults on higher education have led to university boundaries becoming more permeable, so enabling access of those without the traditional qualifications. University curricula have become more flexible, as shown by the development of modular degrees, credit accumulation and transfer systems, the accreditation of prior learning, the provision of franchised courses, open learning and the development of the corporate classroom, all of which are characteristics of a mass system (Scott, 1995). This radical transition from an elite to a mass system attracts little comment from the academic community and the metamorphosis appears to have taken place almost absentmindedly (Daniel, 1993), the point of no return being reached in 1988 when the participation rate for 18/19-year-olds reached 15% (Trow, 1974).

Occupational relevance – the vocational aspects of continuing education

In 1992 parliamentary legislation removed the binary divide between universities and polytechnics, resulting in 158 higher institutions in the UK, of which 90 are now universities (CVCP, 1995). In addition to changing the form of higher education, the State has recently attempted to change its function too by making higher education more vocationally relevant, but this is not the first time that this has happened – there have been State-orchestrated influences on higher education for the last 50 years. For example, the Percy Report of 1945 was the first of these and in the 1950s it led to the establishment of the Colleges of Advanced Technology whose brief was to provide postcompulsory technical education and training. The Robbins Report of 1963 raised the status of certain occupational groups by locating their training in higher education and for the first time vocational qualifications were accepted as a second route of entry to higher education (Smithers and Robinson, 1995). Vocational degrees such as the BTech came into being alongside a range of applied degrees designed as preparation for work in the technical and vocational spheres. Indeed, this trend is evident in the recent history of nurse education and training, with its origin in a work-based apprenticeship model, which later became professionalized (Johnson, 1972) by gaining access and transferring to higher education.

In the 1960s and early 1970s the State (when applying the Robbins principles) provided the resources for the development of a vocational stream in higher education (mainly in the polytechnics) but it did not prescribe how the resources were to be used in the development of curricula. At that time vocational curricula were devised by higher education in collaboration with professional bodies and other occupational groups. Although these curricula were meant to be work-related, a study by Brennon and McGeever (1988) showed that many polytechnic and college graduates considered that they had not been given sufficient opportunities to develop work-related skills on their degrees. State intervention into the prescription of the content of higher education curricula did not take place until the 1980s, after vocational reforms had been introduced into both secondary and further education (Skillbeck, 1994). Skillbeck argues that this direct state intervention into the functions of education was a break with the past: prior to this British governments had always adopted a *laissez-faire* attitude to vocational education and training and in the main had left employers to get on with it themselves. Because of this discontinuity, Skillbeck has called the directive measures 'the new vocationalism'.

The ways and means used to effect vocationalism and occupational relevance in higher education took many forms during a developmental phase. There were specially funded projects, such as the Enterprise in Higher Education initiative (EHEI) for undergraduates and the PICKUP initiative for continuing education students (PICKUP was an acronym for Professional, Industrial and Commercial Knowledge Updating) and the Open Tech. Grants were available from the (then) Manpower Services Commission for training programmes, such as 'Wider Opportunities for Women' and for graduate technical training by means of higher national technology training. Other examples were the more generous levels of funding for degrees that were vocationally relevant.

By the end of the 1980s and in the early 1990s, the government had brought in additional measures designed to increase further the influence of vocationalism on higher education, principally by giving power to employers to influence the curriculum. The first of these measures was a national framework for vocational qualifications, to be overseen by the National Council for Vocational Qualifications (NCVQ), whose membership is drawn from employers and others in industry, commerce and the professions. In 1991, the NCVQ's remit was extended to include first-degree level work and beyond. Another measure arose from the Education Reform Act of 1988, which gave employers and industrialists the opportunity directly to influence universities through their representation on government funding bodies and on the governing bodies of (then) polytechnics, which later became the 'new' universities. A further example is provided by the Training and Enterprise Councils (TECs) whose origins can be traced to the White Paper *Employment for 1990s* (DES, 1988) and which are now operational throughout the UK. The TECs are managed by local employers and businesses and their remit is to administer government training schemes and to encourage and develop training to stimulate local business and enterprise. Their funding depends to some extent on the achievement of output targets such as the delivery of NVQs. In March 1996, TECs were required, for the first time, to have in place procedures for liaison with local higher education providers. As a final example of direct curriculum intervention, part-time adult liberal courses in higher education were mainstreamed after a national consultation and review and, in effect, these programmes were encouraged to become part-time routes on to traditional degree programmes (Duke and Taylor, 1994).

Latterly the State's role has shifted to control of the outputs by means of overarching procedures that act as yardsticks for the quality of higher education provision. Included in these measures are criteria for occupational relevance and institutional response to the needs of employers. These latter two measures are recommended in the report of the National Committee of Inquiry into Higher Education (Dearing, 1997) and, if the State continues along the route set by the historical trends outlined here, these recommendations are likely to be accepted. This chapter was written before the Labour government has indicated how it will respond to the National Committee's report.

In addition to the Dearing Inquiry, the government has set up a task group whose brief includes identifying the future directions for adult education and training. The task group's findings will be fed into a White Paper, which will shape future development for adult/continuing education and training (Fryer, 1997).

THE MARKET – ADULT LEARNERS

In higher education, continuing education courses are generally fee-based so the adults who pay for them can be regarded as customers. About 3.5 million adult customers enrol in formal, organized education each year in the UK (Maguire *et al.*, 1993) and this represents between 10% and 15% of the adult population. About three-quarters of job-related training in Britain is provided by employers outside the formal system (Training Agency, 1989), the remaining quarter taking place in colleges and higher education institutions. Adults enrol on educational courses for a variety of reasons, and any one individual may have several reasons for doing so (NIACE, 1993). Nonetheless, the following four overlapping categories are often used to describe adults in continuing higher education:

- the deferred beginners, who for a variety of reasons start their studies later than is traditional;
- the returners, whose aim is to change their career or life direction after a period of paid work or domestic responsibilities;
- enrichers, whose aims are to know more about things outside their immediate employment;
- developers, who aim to extend their skills and knowledge within the framework of their careers (NIACE, 1993). This last category includes mainly adults on

CPD programmes and, in common with adults in general, their reasons for study are unlikely to be limited solely to updating.

A recent MORI poll (MORI, 1996) has provided some information about the factors that lead adults to engage in learning. When asked for their reasons as to why other people might want to learn something new, 75% of respondents stated work and career reasons. When asked why they themselves wanted to learn new things, they were more likely to say for personal enjoyment (50%) than for work and career reasons (38%). For professionals, the maintenance of technical knowledge and skills appears to be the most important reason (Madden and Mitchell, 1993). In terms of delivery methods adults tend to be rather conservative and state that they learn most from the traditional methods of reading books and other written material (MORI, 1996). This is not surprising, since many returning adults are people who did well in the formal system in their youth (Cross, 1981) and this aspect of conservatism is reflected in Madden and Mitchell's results too (Madden and Mitchell, 1993). Their work shows that the majority of professionals prefer short courses as their first choice for mode of delivery, with journal reading and courses leading to qualifications being second and third choice respectively. When asked who should provide CPD, 80% gave the professional body as the first choice with second choice (65%) being higher education. When choosing CPD, professionals select on the basis of content (90%), cost (50%) and expertise of the presenter (35%). For adult learners in general, the three most commonly cited reasons for non-participation are lack of funding, fear of loss of job security and finding the time to study (McGivney, 1990).

In spite of these barriers to participation, there are many reason why adults will in future continue to demand access to more educational opportunities and there are good reasons for society to enable these demands to be met. Firstly, one of the most important indicators of participation in continuing education is an adult's level of educational attainment – the higher this is on leaving school, the higher the likelihood of demand for participation in later years. In other words, the overall demand is unlikely to go away and governments will be bound to meet these demands and to provide the infrastructures required for social cohesion. Secondly, in societies with an accelerated rate of socioeconomic and technical change, the solutions to attendant problems and the consequent decision-making are provided by adults. The most important learning needs are for those adults currently in the vanguard of change, and international and national economic performance and social well-being depends on their knowledge and wisdom. It is not possible to delay the important decisions facing society in order to wait for young people to grow up and take their place at the helm. A third dimension is a moral one originating in social justice; this has been articulated eloquently by Kennedy (1997), who expresses a widely held view that the development of an individual is a lifelong process and that to deny an individual access to the developmental influences of education is equivalent to deprivation.

Finally, there is an emerging trend of self-directedness, meaning that increasing

numbers of adults are taking responsibility for their own continuing learning. They
are deciding what they want and are 'shopping around' to satisfy these wants and
building up their own bespoke portfolios of learning, rather than accepting the
standardized programmes that are on offer in higher education (Mitchell, 1997).
One barrier to this being a widespread practice has been the lack of a nationally
recognized credit framework but, if and when the Dearing recommendations are
implemented, this practice could become increasingly common. One consequence
of this is as follows. People who take on the design of their own continuing education need to understand how they learn most effectively, and the best place to
learn about this is (arguably) in higher education, where much of our understanding of adult learning has been developed.

Customers as learners: making sense of adult learning

In educational terms, learning generally refers to the process by which changes are
brought about in the way people think, behave and feel. In the process of learning,
people are exposed to new ideas, experiences and roles and inevitably this means
the assimilation of new knowledge. One view of learning is that it is to do with
acquiring knowledge, which is out there, and the learner stores this knowledge in
his/her memory. This view of knowledge has its origins in Western rationality and
has been challenged in recent years by writers such as Guba (1990) whose alternative view is that knowledge is created by the individual as a result of his/her
experience of interacting with and influencing the subject of enquiry. Guba's view
of knowledge means that the learner is not a passive recipient but someone who
has an active role in creating knowledge. The point of all this is that any meaningful discussions about learning need to be preceded by an understanding of how
we view knowledge. The two views given above summarize a complex philosophical debate about the nature of knowledge which is not discussed here in any
depth but is briefly referred to again later in this chapter.

Theoretical models of learning

It is accepted today, almost without question, that adults are capable of learning,
but this was not always believed to be true. Within the field of continuing education there has been a trend for practitioners to rely on findings from psychology
and other disciplines to illuminate their understanding of adult learning The results
of the first systematic attempts in psychology to investigate whether or not adults
could learn were published in 1928 as *Adult Learning* (Thorndike *et al.*, 1928).
Thorndike's work was pioneering because it showed that the ability to keep on
learning did not decrease with age. The importance of Thorndike's approach was
that it was empirical and broke with the tradition of the (then) philosophical
approach of Hobbes, Locke, Hume, Hartley and Mill (Smith, 1987). Thorndike
was part of the 'new psychology' movement, whose model of learning was an
increase in memory. According to this model, memory can be built up step-by-step

and the role of a teacher is to supply the learner with one step after the other, each followed by reward. The origin of this model is in behaviourist psychology, which has many critics but which has influenced formal education in numerous ways and it exists still (for example) in the training and assessment procedures devised for some vocational qualifications, in particular those of the National Council for Vocational Qualifications (NCVQ; Atkins, 1993).

In contrast to the behaviourists, the cognitive psychologists who came later focused their investigations on the information processing aspects of learning. Cognitive models of learning are based on the view that the human brain has a genetically determined mental structure, which varies from one person to another. This mental structure consists of information-processing elements, which can deal with specific types of knowledge, as well as the more general cognitive processes, which differ from one individual to another depending on the individual's prior knowledge, previous experiences and mental structures. The concept of intelligence testing was spawned by this cognitive approach and the idea that there is a single inherited measure of intelligence (Eysenk, 1981) underpins the intelligence quotient (IQ) test. The educational implication of this is that intellect cannot be enhanced much by education, and this is a depressing outlook for most educators. There are numerous critics of the idea that there is a single intelligence factor and, in contrast, Gardiner (1984) argues for seven distinct 'intelligences': linguistic, logical/mathematical, musical, spatial, bodily/kinaesthetic, personal intelligence (concerning other people) and personal intelligence (concerning oneself). The relevance of cognitive psychology to adult learning is that ageing seems to enhance the scores on some aspects of multiple intelligences and worsen the scores on others. The results imply that composite measures of intelligence remain stable until old age.

There is one aspect of cognitive psychology that has commonly been applied to professional education and training: the concept of individual differences in learning. This concept refers to the observable and unquestionable differences in approach and performance shown by each individual in the mastery of learning tasks. The differences are collectively referred to as an individual's 'learning style', which is based on his/her preferences arising from personality, cognitive processing and instructional and environmental influences (Curry, 1987). The purpose of analysing learning styles is (allegedly) to categorize them and use them as a basis for designing education and training programmes, but according to Curry the results of research into learning styles are contentious. Her survey of the literature is inconclusive – learning styles might be artefacts or they might be real enough to be used as the basis for educational planning.

In spite of the ambiguity surrounding learning styles, researchers in the USA have used them to produce applications such as Kolb's learning style inventory (Kolb, 1976) and the Myers–Briggs type indicator (Myers, 1962), both of which are often used in adult training and development programmes. The focus of learning style research in Europe and Australia has been slightly different from the American and has concentrated on detailed observations of groups of learners and the methods they use to approach learning tasks. The most influential workers in this type of study have been Marton and Saljo (1976) and Entwistle and Ramsden (1983) and Entwistle's publication (1992) provides a useful summary. Their studies have indicated that students' approaches to learning can be either 'deep' or 'surface' and an individual can switch according to the nature of the learning task. In other words, the nature of the learning task determines which approach is used, suggesting that an individual's approach is not a fixed entity. Students with a deep orientation are intrinsically motivated and intend to come to grips with a learning task by identifying and understanding its organizing principles; in contrast, the surface orientation is characterized by extrinsic motivation, with the intention of memorizing and reproducing accurately when required. Several other studies indicate the stages through which learners progress as they develop from unskilled novices into experts (see Atkins, 1993 for a brief summary) and Perry's classic work indicates that there are recognizable stages of intellectual development in young adults (Perry, 1970) and that development does not always reach its full potential.

The development of intellectual capacities in adults was once assumed to reach its peak at adolescence, but over the last 20 years attention has turned to the ongoing intellectual and other developments that occur during adulthood. Erikson (1980), Baltes (1987) and others propose models of adult development that refer either to stages in cognitive development (lifespan stages) or to socially determined roles (life course or lifecycle) such as the single adult, the parent, etc. As an example of the socially determined model, Fales (1989) proposes that adult development can pass through nine phases from the late teens through to middle age and old age. During each phase an individual faces certain key problems – for example, in the first adult phase an individual faces the tasks of becoming self-supporting, separating from parents, forming an identity, and so on. This model, although arising from empirical studies, is based on the lives of people living in Western society and for that reason is criticized by Schuller (1992) for its Western orientation and by Caffarella and Olson, who argue that the psychosocial development of women differs from that of men (Caffarella and Olson, 1993).

The earlier dominance of psychology in understanding adult learning was overthrown to some extent by Knowles (1975), who was one of the first practising adult educators to theorize about the ways in which adults learn. He used the term 'andragogy' to encompass the broader aspects of adult learning and to distinguish it from learning in children. Knowles's concept was that adults are self-directed learners, meaning that they tend to take responsibility for their own learning. His principles were (in summary) as follows.

- Adults have a deep psychological need to be self-directing.
- Their experience provides a learning resource.
- Their learning is task- or needs-oriented towards their roles and responsibilities as adults.

- They choose to learn so that they can solve problems rather than learning about a discipline.
- Their learning is intrinsically motivated.

Knowles contrasted these principles with pedagogy (learning in children) and for some time andragogy was regarded as a theory that could be used to underpin the design and delivery of learning programmes for adults. However, the theory of andragogy was eventually undermined by critics who argued that children can be self-directing too. Knowles (1980) later altered his exclusive view of andragogy and now states that self-directed learning is an ideal to which all learners can be encouraged to aspire. There is empirical evidence, provided by Tough's work (1993), that illustrates the self-directedness of one group of adult learners who engage in learning activities outside the formal system principally because their immediate needs are not accommodated by it. The most common motive for these self-directed episodes is the use or application of the acquired knowledge or skill and the least common motive is curiosity about knowledge for its own sake.

Some more recent approaches to understanding adult learning have come from the social constructivists, whose holistic view is that learning is influenced by social and cultural contexts as well as by personal experience and individual history. They argue that learning involves the active participation by the adult learner in his/her construction of meaning from experiences which occur in specific contexts. In other words, new knowledge is created as a product of the interaction between the learner and his/her environment and social context, along the lines of Guba's view of knowledge (Guba, 1990). This means that when adults choose to learn, their motives for learning, what they choose to learn and where they do it are all factors affecting their learning as much as the functioning of their mental processes. In addition, any individual learner is located within society, and society provides some adults with more encouragement and opportunities to learn than others. According to the social constructivists, any understanding of adult learning needs to include the sociological, political and philosophical implications of learning as well as the psychological ones.

These more recent contextual approaches to an understanding of learning (social constructivist) are underpinned by a view of knowledge that contrasts sharply with that held by the first researchers in the psychology of adult learning. Their early behaviourist model of knowledge as quantitative increase in memory has now been replaced by a more complex model incorporating both quantitative and qualitative changes that are subjective and context-related. In spite of the differences between these models they have one element in common, which is that learning involves change. It is the nature of this change that separates one model from the other, and according to Mezirow (1991) much of the theorizing about adult learning is too mechanical and fails to tackle the meaning of this change. He argues that few models can explain how adults make sense of their learning experiences. Mezirow's theory of adult learning attempts to explain meaning and understanding and making sense of experience. It incorporates ideas from a range of disciplines, including philosophy, psychology, social science, neurobiology, linguistics, education and religion. According to his theory, the highest form of learning involves making sense or seeing the full picture of an experience. This form of learning is something that shapes people's lives – they are different afterwards in ways that both they and others can recognize and, according to Mezirow, this is transformational learning and is an ideal towards which all educators of adults should aspire.

Mezirow's work draws heavily on the ideas of Habermas, who believed that human knowledge exists in three distinct domains: technical knowledge relating to the natural world; practical knowledge relating to others and societies; and finally emancipatory knowledge, relating to the self. Habermas argued that, because these knowledge domains are so distinctive, it follows that the methods by which they are learned must be distinctive too.

THE ACADEMIC OLIGARCHY – PROFESSIONAL EDUCATION AND TRAINING WITHIN HIGHER EDUCATION

Universities have a tradition of providing postexperience vocational and professional courses although, as mentioned above, they provide only about 10% of the UK's total, the remainder being provided by employers. University courses may or may not lead to qualifications, and are lumped together collectively as continuing vocational education (CVE). The definition of CVE, according to the Higher Education Funding Council for England (HEFCE, 1996a), is:

> any activity which contributes to the updating of employment-related skills and knowledge to meet the needs of employers and employees (including the self-employed and unemployed). This may include short and long training programmes, CVE related consultancy and research and evaluation of activity.

This all-encompassing definition of CVE includes CPD, which is training for the needs of particular professional groups. In UK universities the term 'continuing vocational education' had its origins in a government funding initiative in 1985 when grants were first made available to some universities to develop postexperience programmes for industry, business, commerce and the professions (Chivers and Nixon, 1993). This government intervention was an example of the new vocationalism in universities (Parker and Richardson, 1996), breaking as it did with the *laissez-faire* attitude of the past and introducing the concept of continuing (as opposed to initial) professional development. This discontinuity has generated a its own vocabulary, according to Barnett (1994), and 'vocationalism' is the new word that has replaced the word 'vocation'. He argues that 'vocation' implies commitment by an individual to a solid base of professional standards and values. In contrast, 'vocationalism' implies adaptability and a rapid response to changes in the world of work. The purpose of vocationalism is to accommodate rapid change and, in contrast, the professional norms and values of a vocation would hinder this adaptability.

CPD is, of course, only part of the vocational education and training of professionals; currently the major part takes place at the initial stage of a professional career (IPD). Although higher education now has a major role in IPD, this was not always the case. The history of the older professions (law, medicine, the Church) is that they developed their own qualifications many years before universities came on the scene and initially they were non-graduate occupations. Later in their history these occupations began to develop a coherent intellectual base and to raise their professional status. They did this through close association with universities, who have increasingly taken on a shared responsibility for their IPD and that of many other professional and occupational groups.

In universities in the UK, the model for the development of the taught curriculum for IPD has been based on cooperation between the professional associations and participating universities and, according to Burrage (1994), the creation of the content of initial professional curricula takes place at the meeting point of two different worlds – that of academia and that of professional practitioners – each of which has different values. University academic curricula value the questioning of received knowledge and the development of individual critical thought and, although these could be at odds with the values of the world of work, Burrage states that public disagreements about the nature of professional curricula are rare. Professional practitioners can act as a conservative brake on innovation in teaching methods or assessment if they perceive change as a lowering of traditional standards, but compromises are generally reached within one of the three models of delivery summarized by Bines (1992). The first is the apprenticeship or pretechnocratic model, which refers mainly to IPD and is delivered mostly on the job but sometimes by block or day release to an educational institution. A second mode of delivery is the technocratic model, which has three main elements, the first being the development of systematic knowledge drawn from the contributing disciplines. The second element is the application of the knowledge base to practice by means of problem-solving and other activities conducted within the context of professional norms and values – the 'nursing process' is an example of this element in nurse education. The third element involves supervision in selected placements. This model generally operates from within an academic institution.

The third delivery model for professional education and training is the posttechnocratic model, which is relatively new and not yet fully developed. According to Bines, this model is increasingly becoming the pattern both for IPD and for CPD. One of its characteristics is the development of professional competencies in practical situations, where trainees are coached by skilled practitioners and are given the opportunities to reflect on their practice. The underpinning disciplines are integrated and learned within the context of professional practice. This model can be located either within an institution or within the workplace or both.

In contrast to IPD, models for the development and delivery of CPD are more varied. Historically, the most common modes of CPD have included compressed events such as conferences, workshops, short courses or slightly longer programmes boosted by distance learning. Professionals also rely on publications in a variety of media, practical experience and other people (Eraut, 1994). The episodic availability of CPD fits in well with the most common learning patterns used by adults: these are short bursts separated by periods of abstention, taking advantage of easily available media. In general, educational coherence is lacking from traditional CPD, mainly because the events are not always organized thematically – they are often isolated, one-off responses to immediate concerns, generated by external events such as changes in legislation, new technology and the like. Another missing element is any linkage between traditional CPD and initial IPD (Eraut, 1994).

As to the purposes of CPD, there is general agreement between the professional bodies and university providers as to what these aims are. The list below indicates the areas of agreement:

- technical or specialist updating relating to professional practice;
- development of new skills in practice;
- interpersonal relationships and social aspects of organizations;
- developing the individual as a continuing, self-directed learner (Madden and Mitchell, 1993; Todd, 1989).

This list provides a historical perspective on CPD curricula and Nowlen (1990) comments on these historical trends, which have moved from a narrow update model to the broader provision of job-related skills (the competence model) and currently to wider coverage of factors, not necessarily job-related, that can affect performance (the holistic or performance model). Mitchell (1997) identifies the beginning of another trend in some professional curricula, namely the introduction of an international perspective, which is particularly apparent in European CPD programmes.

Professional bodies have an additional purpose for CPD as they see it as a means of demonstrating that they are monitoring the continual professional standards of their members (Madden and Mitchell, 1993)

The posttechnocratic model can provide a coherent framework for the delivery of CPD provision but it is not a panacea for the difficulties of selecting appropriate content. Bines's view is that the success of this model rests on the identification of the range of competencies required of an experienced professional. Madden and Mitchell's survey (1993) indicates that, although professional bodies do specify CPD content, the specifications are not necessarily based on their analyses of professional competencies. One currently available analysis of competence resides in NCVQ standards, but the relevance of this as a basis for professional development in higher education is questioned by Hyland (1994) and discussed critically by Eraut (1994). The need to integrate discipline-based knowledge with profession-based knowledge is another problem of content because universities tend to favour discipline-based knowledge whereas practising professionals tend to have the opposite preference. Finally, there is a need to integrate professional workplace practices into the academic curriculum by devising appropriate forms of assessment. According to Portwood (1993, 1996) higher education can address questions of content through work-based learning (WBL). He argues that WBL can be accommodated by higher education but this does require changes in academic systems and procedures. Fulton, McHugh and Saunders (1996) push this argument further by stating that some academics may not be willing or able to deliver WBL, and here lies a problem for CPD practitioners in higher education.

The root of this problem lies in the design and delivery of educational programmes when their aims are translated into the operational activities of planned intentional learning – content, delivery, assessment and evaluation. These are the components of a taught curriculum, each reflecting underpinning ideologies about the nature of knowledge. For CPD, the knowledge base is wide, ranging across a spectrum from technical know-how to interpersonal competencies and then to knowledge about oneself. Without pressing the comparisons too far, it is possible to identify Habermas's three forms of knowledge about the world in the CDP curriculum. If there is any substance to Habermas's ideas, these three forms of knowledge each require distinctive teaching and learning methods and this raises questions about the integrity of the elements of vocationalism – the transferability of skills, adaptability and the integration of academic learning with WBL.

Notwithstanding the distinctions between different forms of knowledge, there are dissimilarities in the methods used to generate knowledge about the world (Usher and Bryant, 1987). They argue that the distinctions between the methods used to create knowledge are important to understand, especially for providers of professional education and training. They argue that formal theoretical knowledge is the form of knowledge generated by higher education. It is based on abstract conceptualizations of the world; its theories are generalizable and may not be testable in specific circumstances. In contrast, practitioner knowledge is generated through direct interaction with the world. It is based on dealing with each situation as it arises and is applicable only to that one situation. Schon (1983) believes that practitioner knowledge has a lower status than formal theoretical knowledge because the latter is traditionally regarded as the fount from which practitioner knowledge springs. According to Schon any links between practice and theory are speculative because problems of practice cannot always be solved by applying theory. He sees professional practice as an area where problems arise (without being predefined) and therefore there are no predetermined ends. The gap between practice and theory is where the professional uses his or her professional judgement, based on previous knowledge and experience and has to change his/her approach according to changing situations which may be influenced by factors outside his/her control. This is a dynamic model in which the relationship between theory and practice is integrated through transaction.

The problem for CPD practitioners in the milieu of higher education is that formal theory is regarded as the norm, and this is reflected in many ways through the cultural values and practices of the academic community. Any attempt to shift the balance away from their norms will be met with resistance. This is a major challenge faced by those in higher education who attempt to develop curricula directly relevant to professional practice.

IMPLICATIONS FOR THE FUTURE

The future pattern of higher education provision in the UK is still developing and this chapter was written just after the publication of the National Committee of Inquiry Report into the future of higher education in the UK (Dearing, 1997). This report is quite clear about the need to involve employers more in higher education and to continue with occupational relevance in university curricula. However, the seeds of the future were already sown before the publication of this report, which essentially has summarized many of the trends apparent in the past two decades. As indicated above, the government has yet to take on board any of the report's recommendations and is currently preparing a White Paper on adult learning.

Whatever happens next is unlikely to be discontinuous with recent historical trends. For example, the state's future policies are likely to continue to encourage both vocationalism and access and these two themes will have implications for continuing education in higher education. One possibility is that access and vocationalism may become closely coupled and consequently any increase in publicly funded access will be linked to vocational provision. As an example, the Labour Party has promised a University for Industry, the aim of this proposal being to increase the supply of higher level (mostly subdegree) work-related training and to make it more accessible (Hillman, 1996). Another possibility is that the state could bring pressure to bear on the curriculum of higher education in general so that it becomes closely geared to the perceived requirements for trained personnel. The means of operating this pressure is unlikely to be direct curricular intervention but more probably externally imposed, national evaluative frameworks – in other words, through a quality assurance framework that selectively rewards vocational elements in the curriculum. Dearing's qualifications framework provides an opportunity to do this.

Alongside these measures to intensify the vocational focus of higher education, private funding from a variety of sources is likely to be encouraged, including student fees. Already the government has accepted the principle of introducing tuition fees for full-time undergraduates, arguing that this brings them into line with part-time students, who have always paid a fee. This, coupled with measures to introduce loans for maintenance grants, sets a new agenda for the privatization of higher education. Privatization occurs also when firms (such as Ford) buy bespoke training programmes and degrees from universities and there are already many examples of this type of provision.

Public funding for part-time students (via loans) seems at present not to be an option because of the prohibitive expense. However, across the regions of the UK, public funding (originating from government) is directed through numerous channels and agencies (the TECs, the LEAs, etc.) into education and training. By forming liaisons and partnerships with these agencies, universities can harvest some of the resources of a shrinking public purse, but these liaisons can diminish the autonomy that is so precious to higher education. This autonomy is manifest in the design and delivery of curricula, and when they are being paid for through a complex partnership, curricula generally need to demonstrate the interests of all partners, some of whom are likely to be vocationally oriented. Ironically, some employers are prepared to provide employees with financial assistance towards studies of their own choice, preferably courses that are not work-related (Moore, 1994).

In the same way as access to first-degree level was an issue for the previous two decades, access by non-graduate mid-career professionals to postexperience/postgraduate level will be an issue for the future. Alternative modes of entry based on the recognition of experiential learning will be needed to accommodate the demands from these fee-paying students, whose economic potential will be very attractive to institutions. The concept of a Learning Bank to encourage individuals to invest long-term is an option that is still on the political agenda (e.g. Robertson, 1995) but whose fate has not yet been decided. However, the notion of lifetime or lifelong learning is now supported by the State, on the understanding that each individual will be responsible for organizing and paying for his/her own. There are many implications surrounding this privatization of higher education, not least its inequity, the influence of the 'purchasers' on the curriculum and the possibilities of litigation when customers receive unsatisfactory provision.

If higher education is to survive in this new world, it will need to accommodate the needs of new cohorts of students whose requirements will be for flexible and accessible learning opportunities that they can fit into busy schedules. Lifelong learning for professionals can best be enhanced by developing a continuum between IPD and CPD by introducing learners at an early stage into the concept of learning to learn and by using the best practices gleaned from those who have expertise in adult learning. What is needed for the design and delivery of high-quality professional programmes is support and guidance to enable learners to construct their own path through a coherent programme of learning, which may be drawn from disparate providers (the employer, the professional body and higher education) and delivered in different modes. Providers of CPD will need to market to professional bodies, practitioners and employers, bearing in mind that for those who pay for themselves the cost is likely to be a significant factor, whereas this is not necessarily the case for some large private sponsors.

CPD providers in higher education will inevitably be affected by the differentiation that is becoming apparent within the UK's mass system of higher education, with some more affluent universities attempting to place themselves in an exclusive league at the top of an increasingly stratified system (Scott, 1995). Consequently some CPD providers might find themselves in rarefied positions as centres of excellence based either on the reputation of their institution or on themselves as providers. To sustain this position they will need to generate increasing amounts of private income by reaching more clients through increasingly diverse modes of delivery such as open and distance learning, delivering in-company and in collaboration with private and other providers using the flexible, modular programmes and assessment methods characteristic of a mass system.

For continuing educators, one important future role is to disseminate widely within higher education the principles and practice of high-quality education for adults. Adults as learners in higher education are located in a system geared to the needs of young, full-time students and in many respects the system operates as if it were still an elite (Daniel, 1993). This works in opposition to the needs as learners of adults, who have a wider range of ages, attitudes, goals, settings and learning styles than do young people and who choose to be engaged continually in some form of learning, either as part of everyday life or within the formal, organized system.

For an educational system that aims to enhance lifelong learning, there are operational implications in focusing on how adults learn and these are as follows. Firstly, adults rely on short learning episodes that are interspersed with everyday events and are focused on their interests or curiosity about specific issues. Consequently, content needs to be relevant and focused on specific issues that relate new material to what is already known. Secondly, adults generally plan for themselves, so it is important to involve the learners in planning some (or all) of their learning tasks. However, in certain situations directive teaching methods are required: for example, if a person is starting a new subject s/he will need some didactic instruction but when s/he has developed a foundation of knowledge s/he can become more autonomous as a learner.

Thirdly, adult students may well be aware of their preferred styles of learning and so the practitioner needs to use as many different methods as possible to accommodate them. However, students who have progressed successfully through the formal system are most likely to prefer traditional delivery methods and will not necessarily embrace innovation immediately. Fourthly, if adult development theorists are correct, then not all adults have developed to their full intellectual potential but they can be encouraged to do so through the design and delivery of appropriate programmes.

Finally, within the current climate of vocationalism the relevance of formal theory is continually being questioned; continuing educators too question its hold on the curriculum, but for reasons that are associated with the needs of adult learners. The vocational imperative is giving rise to some attempts to link work and academe, through developments that appear to overlook the fundamental differences in their respective knowledge bases and so could be doomed to failure. Is the way forward for CPD the development of practitioner theory? Practitioner theory could lead to the development of professionals who embrace theoretical rules but whose self-confidence prepares them to abandon these rules when appropriate in favour of trusting their own experience. This is the essence of a self-directed learner and, as well as developing the individual, it could also lead to greater effectiveness in practice. Here lies a real challenge for all those interested in the continuing education of adults.

REFERENCES

Aldcroft, D. H. (1992) *Education, Training and Economic Performance, 1944 to 1990*, Manchester University Press, Manchester.

Atkins, M. (1993) *Assessment Issues in Higher Education*, Department of Employment, Sheffield.

Baltes, P. (1987) Theoretical propositions of life-span development psychology. *Developmental Psychology*, **23**, 611–626.

Barnett, R. (1994) *The Limits of Competence. Knowledge, Higher Education and Society*, Society for Research into Higher Education and Open University Press, Buckingham.

Benn, R. and Fieldhouse, R. (1993) Government policies on university expansion and wider access, 1945 and 1985 compared. *Studies in Higher Education*, **18**(3), 299–313.

Bines, H. (1992) Issues in course design, in *Developing Professional Education*, (eds H. Bines and D. Watson), Society for Research into Higher Education and Open University Press, Buckingham.

Brennon, J. and McGeever, P. (1988) *Graduates at Work; Degree Course and the Labour Market,* Jessica Kingsley, London.

Burrage, M. (1994) Routine and discreet relationships: professional education and the State in Britain, in *Governments and Professional Education*, (ed. T. Becher), Society for Research into Higher Education and Open University Press, Buckingham, pp. 140–158.

Caffarella, R. S. and Olson, S. K. (1993) Psychosocial development of women: a critical review of the literature. *Adult Education Quarterly*, **43**(3), 125–151.

Chivers, G. and Nixon, N. (1993) *PICKUP in Universities*, Division of Adult Continuing Education, University of Sheffield, Sheffield.

Clark, B. (1983) *Higher Education Systems. Academic organisation in cross-national perspectives,* University of California Press, Berkeley, CA.

Cross, P. (1981) *Adults as Learners: Increasing Participation and Facilitating Learning*, Jossey-Bass, San Francisco, CA.

Curry, L. (1987) *Integrating Concepts of Cognitive or Learning Style: A Review with Attention to Psychometric Standards*, Canadian College of Health Service Executives, Ottawa.

CVCP (1995) *Higher Education Statistics Autumn 1995,* Committee of Vice-Chancellors and Principals, London.

Dale, R. (1989) What is the State? in *The State and Education Policy*, Open University Press, Milton Keynes, pp. 53–57.

Daniel, J. (1993) The challenge of mass higher education. *Studies in Higher Education*, **18**(2), 197–203.

Davies, G. (1995) *The Role of the Higher Education Funding Councils and their Support for CVE*, UACE, University of Lancaster, Lancaster.

Dearing, R. (1997) *Higher Education in the Learning Society – Reports 5 and 6*, National Committee of Inquiry into Higher Education, Stationery Office, Norwich.

DES (1988) *Student Numbers in Higher Education: Great Britain 1975–1986*, Statistical Bulletin, August, HMSO, London.

Duke, C. and Taylor, R. (1994) The HEFCE review and the funding of continuing education. *Studies in the Education of Adults*, **26**(1), 86–94.

Entwistle, N. (1992) *The Impact of Teaching on Learning Outcomes in Higher Education*, Committee of Vice-Chancellors and Principals (Staff Development Unit), Sheffield.

Entwistle, N. J. and Ramsden, P. J. (1983) *Understanding Student Learning*, Croom Helm, London.

Eraut, M. (1994) *Developing Professional Knowledge and Competence*, Falmer Press, London.

Erikson, E. H. (1980) *Identity and the Life-cycle: A Reissue*, Norton, New York.

Eysenk, H. J. (1981) *The Intelligence Controversy*, John Wiley, New York.

Fales, A.W. (1989) Life-span learning development, in *Lifelong Education for Adults: An International Handbook*, (ed. C. J. Titmus), Pergamon Press, Oxford, pp. 183–187.

Fryer, W. (1997) Tasks, time-scales and ways of working. *Adults Learning*, **9**(1), 6–7.

Fulton, O., McHugh, G. and Saunders, M. (1996) *Work-based Learning and its Accreditation: Can Higher Education Deliver?*, Centre for the Study of Education and Training, Lancaster University, Lancaster.

Gardiner, H. (1984) *Frames of Mind: The Theory of Multiple Intelligence*, Heinemann, London.

Guba, E. (1990) *The Paradigm Dialogue,* Sage, Newbury Park, CA.

Halsey, A.H. (1993) Trends in access and equity in higher education: Britain in international perspective. *Oxford Review of Higher Education*, **19**(2), 129–140.

HEFCE (1996a) Continuing Vocational Education (CVE) development funding: monitoring of 1995–96 academic year. *Circular 14/96*, Higher Education Funding Council for England, Bristol.

HEFCE (1996b) *Widening Access to Higher Education. A Report by the HEFCE's Advisory Group on Access and Participation,* Higher Education Funding Council, Bristol.

Hillman, J. (1996) *University for Industry. Creating a National Learning Network*, Institute for Public Policy Research, Lincoln.

Hore, T. (1993) Non-traditional students. Third-age and part-time, in *The Encyclopaedia of Higher Education*, (eds B. R. Clark and G. Neave), Pergamon Press, Oxford.

Hyland, T (1994) Experiential learning, competence and critical practice in higher education. *Studies in Higher Education*, **19**(3), 327–339.

Johnson, T. L. (1972) *Professions and Power*, Macmillan, London.

Kennedy, H. (1997) *Learning Works. Widening Participation in Further Education*, Further Education Funding Council, Coventry.

Knowles, M. S. (1975) *Self-Directed Learning*, Association Press, New York.

Knowles, M. S. (1980) *The Modern Practice of Adult Education: From Pedagogy to Andragogy*, 2nd edn, Cambridge Books, New York.

Kolb, D. (1976) *Learning Style Inventory Technical Manual*, McBer & Co., Boston, MA.

Maguire, M., Maguire, S. and Felstead, A. (1993) *Factors Influencing Individual Commitment to Lifetime Learning. A Literature Review*, Department of Employment, Sheffield.

Madden, C.A. and Mitchell, V.A. (1993) *Professions, Standards and Competence*, Department of Continuing Education, University of Bristol.

Marton, F. and Saljo, R. (1976) On qualitative differences in learning. *British Journal of Educational Psychology*, **46**, 4–11.

McGivney, V. (1990) *Access to Education for Non-Participant Adults*, National Institute for Adult and Continuing Education, Leicester.

Mezirow, J. (1991) *Transformative Dimensions of Adult Learning*, Jossey-Bass, San Francisco, CA.

Mitchell, M. (1997) Continuing professional development challenges for the professions in

Europe. Keynote address, Continuing Vocational Education Annual Conference, University of York, September.

Moore, R. (1994) Ford EDAP. *Adults Learning*, **5**(9), 225–226.

MORI (1996) *State of the Nation Poll*, MORI, London.

Myers, I.B. (1962) *The Myers–Briggs Type Indicator*, Consulting Psychologists Press, Palo Alto, CA.

NIACE (1993) *An Adult Higher Education*, National Institute for Adult and Continuing Education, Leicester.

Nowlen, P.M. (1990) New expectations, new roles: a holistic approach to continuing education for the professions, in *Visions for the Future of Continuing Professional Education*, (eds R. M. Cervero *et al.*), University of Georgia, Athens, GA.

Parker, S. and Richardson, M. (1996) Continuing Vocational Education: the role of PICKUP funding, in *Continuing Education in the Mainstream: The Funding Issues, UACE Occasional Paper 17*, (eds R. Taylor and D. Watson), Universities Association for Continuing Education, University of Warwick, Warwick, pp. 51–61.

Parry, G. (1995) England, Wales and Northern Ireland, in *International Perspectives on Access and Participation*, (ed. P. Davies), Jessica Kingsley, London, pp. 102–133.

Perry, W. G. (1970) *Forms of Intellectual and Ethical Development in the College Years: A Scheme*, Holt, Rinehart & Winston, New York.

Portwood, D. (1993) Work based learning: linking academic and vocational qualifications. *Journal of Further and Higher Education*, **17**(3), 61–69.

Portwood, D. (1996) *An Overview of Work-based Learning in Higher Education. Has it a Future?*, University of Middlesex, London.

Robertson, D. (1995) *The Learning Bank. Towards a Strategy for Investment in Post-compulsory Education and Training*, John Moores University, Liverpool.

Schon, D. (1983) *The Reflective Practitioner: How Professionals Think in Action*, Basic Books, New York.

Schuller, T. (1992) Age, gender and learning in the life-span, in *Learning Across the Life-span: Theories, Research, Policies*, (eds A. C. Tuijnam and M. van der Kamp), Pergamon Press, Oxford, pp. 17–32.

Scott, P. (1995) *The Meanings of Mass Higher Education*, Society for Research into Higher Education and Open University Press, Buckingham.

Skillbeck, M., Connell, H., Lowe, N. and Tait, R. (1994) *The Vocational Quest: New Directions in Education and Training*, Routledge, London.

Smith, W.A. (1987) E. L. Thorndike, in *Twentieth Century Thinkers in Adult Education*, (ed. P. Jarvis), Routledge, London.

Smithers, A. and Robinson, P. (1995) *Post-18 Education: Growth, Change, Prospect*, Council for Industry and Higher Education, London.

Thorndike, E. L., Bregman, E. O., Tilton, J. W. and Woodyard, E. (1928) *Adult Learning*, Macmillan, New York.

Todd, F. (1989) Learning and work: directions for continuing professional and vocational education. *International Journal of Lifelong Education*, **3**(2), 89–104.

Tough, A. (1993) Self-planned learning and major personal change, in *Adult Learners, Education and Training*, (eds R. Edwards, S. Sieminski and D. Zeldin), Routledge, in association with the Open University, London, pp. 31–41.

Training Agency (1989) *Training in Britain: A Study of Funding, Activities and Attitudes – The Main Report*, Training Agency, Sheffield.

Trow, M. (1974) Problems in the transition from elite to mass higher education, in *Organization for Economic Co-operation and Development Policies for Higher Education*, Organization for Economic Co-operation and Development, Paris.

Usher, R. and Bryant, I. (1987) Re-examining the Theory–Practice Relationship. *Studies in Higher Education*, **12**(2), 201–211.

Watts, B. (1996) Continuing professional education in England and Wales, in *European Manual of Continuing Education*, Luchterland, Sonderruck.

5

Planning the NHS workforce – the role of professional development

Philip Gill

INTRODUCTION

The National Health Service is the largest civilian employer in Europe, employment in the NHS accounting for almost 780 000 in 1993 (OPCS, 1995). Given the scale of employment it is right and proper for detailed consideration to be given to understanding this workforce, how it is composed, what trends are emerging in relation to it and the costs associated with it.

The past few years have seen an increasing emphasis on the importance of good and innovative approaches to planning and managing this workforce. As will be discussed later, there have been significant developments in approaches to such planning and understanding, especially since the creation of the NHS 'internal market' in 1991.

This chapter will seek to map out some of the main issues associated with NHS workforce planning in general and in relation to the nursing workforce in particular. In doing so the following structure will be adopted. After a consideration of the scope of the NHS workforce, including an understanding of employment patterns, and the particular situation facing the nursing workforce, there will be a consideration of why planning has been seen to be of greater importance in the 1990s by examining a range of factors that have impacted on both the supply and demand for staff within the NHS. Following this will be an overview of how the NHS currently plans for its workforce and a discussion of the challenges that the new approaches face. Moving on from this discussion, the literature relating to 'manpower planning' and the newer term 'strategic human resource planning' will be discussed and put in the context of the NHS workforce, from which a range of developments will be proposed, many of which currently form best practice within the NHS. Central to these developments will be a discussion of the concept of career and the 'new deal' in employment relationships. This will then link into a discussion of the role that professional development will need to take in developing these new employment relationships. Finally, the chapter concludes with some policy considerations for the new education and training consortia if professional development is to take a more proactive role in workforce planning.

THE SCOPE OF THE NHS WORKFORCE

Figure 5.1 shows the NHS workforce for England as at 30 September 1994.

Staff group	n
Medical and dental*	52 153
Nursing and midwifery†	353 128
Professions allied to medicine	40 475
Professional and technical	37 901
Scientific and professional	14 392
Works professional	2760
Maintenance (building and engineering)	12 438
General and senior managers	22 954
Administrative and clerical	134 610
Ambulance officers and control assistants	2543
Ambulance men/women	15 406
Ancillary	72 816
Others‡	1380
Total	762 956

* Figures include locum and agency locum staff

† Figures include agency staff and health visitor students but exclude students on Project 2000 courses (around 32 000 in 1994)

‡ A change in data collection procedures in 1991 resulted in the 'other' category representing health care assistants (HCAs) and other staff on locally determined pay – a further change in 1993 resulted in most of these others being recategorized into the main staff groups

Figure 5.1 The NHS workforce in 1994 in England (as at 30 September 1996); figures for directly employed staff are in whole-time equivalents (Wte) – the total number of hours worked divided by the basic hours per grade and staff group (source: Government Statistical Service, 1996)

These figures clearly show the importance to the health service of nursing staff, this being the largest staff group and representing 46.3% of the NHS workforce in England (separate statistics are collected for Scotland, Wales and Northern Ireland by the Scottish, Welsh and Northern Ireland offices respectively). What is, however, more interesting is to examine the nursing numbers over a period of time (Figure 5.2) and the numbers and percentage 'economically active' and in employment (Figure 5.3).

Year	Wte (%)
1983	397 100 (47.8%)
1986	402 700 (50.2%)
1987	404 000 (50.5%)
1988	403 900 (50.9%)
1989	405 300 (50.9%)
1990	402 100 (50.5%)
1991	396 100 (49.5%)
1992	382 000 (48.0%)
1993	366 200 (47.3%)
1994	353 100 (46.3%)

Figure 5.2 The NHS nursing workforce (England) 1983–1994 – whole-time equivalents (Wte) and percentage of the workforce (source: Government Statistical Service, 1996)

Region	All (000s)	Economically active (000s)	In employment (000s)
UK	675	560 (83%)	554 (82%)
Great Britain	651	541 (83%)	536 (82%)
South-east	190	153 (80%)	150 (79%)
East Anglia	27	21 (79%)	21 (79%)
South-west	59	51 (85%)	51 (85%)
West Midlands	53	45 (85%)	45 (85%)
Yorkshire and Humberside	52	44 (84%)	43 (83%)
North-west	78	65 (84%)	65 (84%)
North	35	30 (86%)	29 (85%)
Wales	41	35 (86%)	35 (86%)
Scotland	66	56 (86%)	55 (83%)
Northern Ireland	24	18 (77%)	18 (77%)

Figure 5.3 The tight labour market for nurses: economic activity of people of working age whose highest qualification is nursing, spring 1996; 'economically active' includes individuals in or seeking work (source: Department of Employment, 1996)

Figure 5.2 shows an increase in the size of the nursing workforce over the period 1983–1989 but a steady reduction from 1990 onwards. This has been high-lighted by professionals and politicians as a cause for concern and has been con-trasted, in particular, with a significant rise in the number of general and senior managers over the same period (from 500 in 1986 to almost 23 000 in 1994). More interestingly, this reduction has occurred at the same time as the NHS is experi-encing rising activity levels and rising patient dependency, and at a time when increasing numbers of nurses are to be found working in private nursing homes, the independent sector and GP practices.

This last point may go some way to explaining the data in Figure 5.3, which draws on Department of Employment Labour Force Survey data. This shows that, of the total number of individuals of a working age in the UK with nursing as their highest qualification, 83% are economically active (in work or seeking work) and 82% are in employment. This suggests that, while the nursing reduction evident in Figure 5.2 has not led to significant pools of unemployed nurses, the numbers available to enter the workforce, should demand for staff increase, are very small. The Institute of Employment Studies (IES, 1996) estimates that there are not many more than 20 000 nurses available to return to nursing employment. One probable reason for this is that a number of individuals who have nursing as their highest qualification have moved into other spheres of employment, be they other 'caring' roles or more commercial roles. Nevertheless, the position still exists that there is no large 'pool' of nurses available to the NHS to meet any increases in demand for staff. This is of particular concern since there is growing evidence that demand is indeed increasing. Such evidence can be gauged from the Office of Manpower Economics (reported in IES, 1996), which is recording an increasing number of nursing vacancies as unfilled, and the 1996 report of the Pay Review Body for Nursing Staff, Midwives and Professions Allied to Medicine (Review Body, 1996). All of this evidence seems to point to an increasing imbalance between the demand for and supply of nursing staff.

Traditionally, at times of such imbalances the NHS has increased the number of places it offers to students wishing to study to become nurses. The Institute of Employment Studies report (IES, 1996) found, however, that between 1987/88 and 1994/95 the size of the intake to preregistration nurse education had dropped by 39%. These reductions were confirmed by falling levels of new entries on the reg-ister of the United Kingdom Central Council for Nursing, Midwifery and Health Visiting (UKCC).

While there is evidence that the number of training places being commissioned in 1996/97 and 1997/98 is 14% higher than in 1995/96 (IES, 1996) the effect of this will not be felt until 2000, given the 3-year duration of the education course. Thus at a macro level the possibility of a continued imbalance between the supply of nursing staff and the demand for such staff remains. But what are the reasons for the increasing demand for such staff and what trends can be identified within the current nursing workforce (current supply) that may affect the situation further?

SUPPLY AND DEMAND FOR NURSING STAFF

When considering the supply and demand for nursing staff within the NHS and the wider health-care sector it is important to realize that a range of factors will be relevant to each individual provider of health care and may differ from other such organizations. There are, however, a range of general trends that have impacted on health services over the last few years which will, in part, provide some insights as to why an imbalance exists between the demand for and supply of nurses.

General factors impacting on workforce demand and supply

Demographics

In the late 1980s the NHS was warned of a 'demographic time-bomb' (Conroy and Stidson, 1988): the reduction in the number of school leavers in the 1990s would, it was argued, leave the NHS extremely vulnerable given its reliance on new recruits. However, this report could not foresee the global economic recession of the late 1980s and early 1990s. The effect of this recession was to seriously reduce other employment sectors that might have been expected to recruit from the tradi- tional NHS recruitment pool of school leavers with five or more GCSEs. As a result of this the potential supply of new recruits was not as small as was feared. However, the recession did affect the NHS workforce in another way. The impact of the recession on public finances constrained public expenditure on the NHS. As a result, many employers did not recruit in traditional numbers and also sought to replace perceived 'high-cost' professional staff with lower-cost 'support workers', a move that some called a 'de-skilling' of the NHS workforce (Bagust, Burrows and Oakley, 1992).

More recently, however, we have seen other elements of the demographic dimension impact on the supply of and demand for nursing staff. Firstly the 'age- ing' population identified by Conroy and Stidson (1988) has greatly influenced the demand for health services as the dependency of the population has increased. Secondly 'female participation rates' - the number of females in the workforce – have always been high within the NHS (Corby (1991) estimated that 90% of the nursing workforce is female) and there is evidence that in the late 1990s these female workers expect work to be better organized to meet their needs. The IES (1996) estimated that the caring responsibilities of many of the nursing workforce were very high (41% responsible for dependent children, 16% responsible for dependent adults, 4% for both). Unless the NHS responds to these needs in terms of how work is organized it is likely that a sizeable number of nurses with these responsibilities will seek work with more appropriate working patterns. Thirdly, as the recession lifts the other employment sectors that compete with the NHS for school leavers are likely to become more active in the labour market, thereby increasing pressure on the NHS in terms of its ability to attract new recruits.

Finally, without significant numbers of new recruits the nursing workforce will age, with the likelihood of greater numbers of retirements increasing demand further (IES, 1996).

Structural change and central government initiatives

The creation of the NHS internal market represented a massive change in the organization and management of health services. Inevitably, this has had a significant impact on the nursing workforce. The full extent of these changes has been discussed fully elsewhere (see, for example, Robinson and Le Grand, 1994). However, a few examples of the impact on the demand for and supply of nurses are provided below.

Efficiency and effectiveness

Value for money has been at the heart of many of the NHS reforms; this has impacted on staff demand in a number of ways. The quest for yet more efficiency savings has led many health-care providers to seek to replace professional staff with support workers. The impact on nursing has often been quite dramatic, with many providers seeking to rebalance the ratio between qualified and unqualified staff. Often this has been driven by supposed 'one best way' methodologies (see, for example, NHS Management Executive Value for Money Unit, 1990). At the same time this quest for efficiency has led to many management roles being created at local and ward level, with the result that significant numbers of nurses are now classified as senior managers, altering the statistics of nursing numbers even further.

The quest for continuing efficiency and effectiveness is likely to have had a more subtle impact on the supply of nurses. According to the IES survey (1996) 23% of nurses questioned cited 'dissatisfaction with job' as the reason for leaving the NHS. While dissatisfaction may stem from many sources it is likely that reorganization and efficiency savings have some impact on this. This point will be developed further when we look at how workforce planning within the NHS may develop and how professional development will affect this.

Changes in the medical workforce

The NHS medical workforce is undergoing some significant changes as a result of central initiatives, many of which will have a direct impact on nursing demand and the types of role required. Two key initiatives are the 'new deal for junior doctors' (Department of Health, 1991) and the Calman Report on the future specialist training of medical staff (Department of Health, 1993). These two reports have, and will continue to have, a profound impact on doctors in training but will also impact on other health-care professionals, especially nurses. Taken together, the reduction in hours worked and contracted (the New Deal) and the reduced length of and more formal teaching in specialist training will mean that a whole range of duties traditionally performed by medical staff will need to be undertaken by other staff groups within the NHS. Early in the implementation of the 'New Deal' there was some evidence from regional task forces (charged with ensuring implementation of proposals) that tasks were 'dumped' on other staff groups. However, more recently there is evidence that both initiatives are being implemented in a more measured way with 'appropriate' tasks and roles being taken on by other staff (see, for example, Greenhalgh and Co., 1994, and Meadows, 1997). The increasing numbers of specialist nursing roles and nurse practitioners can in part be attributed to the implementation needs of these two initiatives. It is highly likely that, as a result of the emergence of these roles, the boundaries between doctors and nurses, and nurses and other professional and support staff, will continue to be challenged and will influence nursing demand.

Changes in technology and the philosophy of care

Technological advances continue to greatly influence health-care practice. Part of the reason for increasing demand for nursing specialists is to be able to respond to these advances and use new techniques, treatments and procedures to improve patient care. Clearly this is an area where the availability of professional development is crucial. However, as well as creating opportunities for developing more specialist roles there is the possibility that technology may replace certain tasks or make them more appropriate to other staff groups.

Technological advances are also evident in the way health care and health services are being organized and reorganized in the 1990s, with approaches such as 'patient-centred care' and 'hospital process re-engineering' (see Oram and Wellins, 1995, for an NHS example) becoming more widespread. Behind these approaches are new philosophies of care that seek to organize health services around the needs of patients rather than managerial or physical boundaries. The reasons for adopting these approaches are debatable, the cost pressures facing NHS providers being cited as many times as new philosophies of care. The important point is that where these projects are being undertaken there is significant impact on the design of jobs and roles to meet the requirements of new ways of working that will potentially alter the demand for staff, nurses included.

Staff turnover and wastage

As well as the strategic and demographic factors outlined above it is important to understand that the supply and demand imbalance within the nursing workforce is also influenced by turnover and wastage among current staff. The IES report (1996) recorded that for the third consecutive year turnover among nurses within the NHS had risen (from 15% in 1993/94 to 22% in 1995/96 – although this masks regional variations of up to 36%). While much of this turnover can be explained by nurses moving from one NHS provider to another (traditionally from NHS trust to trust, but now just as likely to be from trust to primary care provider), this cannot be cause for comfort since wastage (the number of nurses leaving the NHS) has risen over the same 3-year period from 4% to 6%. With a nursing workforce in England of 353 000 this represents a loss in 1995/96 of just over 21 000 nurses. As well as impacting on the availability of staff this situation has severe financial consequences, since the Audit Commission (1997) has calculated that the average cost of replacing three 'E' grade nurses (a typical recruitment exercise) is £4900.

A degree of staff turnover and wastage is considered to be a good thing. The Audit Commission (1997) argued that turnover and wastage can allow 'new blood' to join the organization and present opportunities for restructuring. However, continuity of care, retention of expertise and costs are negative factors. For those health-care providers that are experiencing high turnover (especially up to the 36% mentioned earlier) the costs involved in replacing staff must run into tens of thousands of pounds.

Reasons why nurses leave the employment of one organization for another must be of concern to practitioners and policy-makers alike. The IES survey (1996) shows 23% leaving because of job dissatisfaction and 24% leaving to acquire new skills; the Audit Commission provided supporting evidence to these figures by stating that more than half the variation between NHS trusts with high and low turnover can be explained by differences in how trusts manage their staff. As a result, it is clear that these are factors that many providers can influence and their approaches to doing so will be discussed in some detail later in this chapter.

Having looked in general at some of the factors that impact on the supply and demand for nursing staff, specifically within the NHS but applicable to other health-care providers, it follows that the NHS workforce planning process should take account of these factors in developing local and national approaches to workforce planning. To begin with, however, it is important to understand the NHS workforce planning system and how it has developed in recent times.

WORKFORCE PLANNING IN THE NHS

Prior to the creation of the NHS internal market in 1991 most workforce planning relating to non-medical staff had been conducted in a rather parochial way. Each regional health authority had well-staffed 'manpower planning' departments (the term 'workforce planning' more accurately reflects the situation, given that 70% of the NHS workforce is female!). These departments conducted wide-ranging studies looking at the characteristics of the workforce, trends that were emerging and predicted supply and demand over long periods of time. Equally, education and training was provided in the same parochial way, with the NHS having 'in-house' training schools within a number of district health authorities. This set of circumstances meant that workforce planning received little serious attention, especially since the large sums of money being spent were essentially hidden within district health authorities' overall financial accounting systems (Humphreys, 1994).

With the introduction of the 1991 NHS reforms (Department of Health, 1990) this funding situation needed to change, since a key principle of the act was to focus on funding and costing health care directly rather than other 'peripheral' activities such as education. The mechanism to achieve this was initially outlined in the original White Paper that trailed the reforms, *Working for Patients* (Department of Health, 1989a), and more specifically, a working paper attached to this White Paper regarding education and training, colloquially known as 'Working Paper 10' (Department of Health, 1989b). Working Paper 10 established two key principles with regard to education and training: firstly, the direct funding of education and training via regional health authorities (RHAs) and secondly, the devolution of workforce planning responsibilities to local NHS providers (usually NHS trusts and, in the early days of the arrangements, directly managed units).

For the first year or two of these new relationships efforts appeared to focus on two key areas from the RHA perspective: firstly, to try and ensure that the funding arrangements worked smoothly, which in itself was a major effort, and secondly, to try and improve workforce planning at local, NHS trust level. Trusts and directly managed units were required to produce workforce planning statements that forecast the numbers of staff they would need over a future period of time for each staff group. These statements were passed to RHAs, who 'validated' this information. This validation exercise was a contentious issue since some trusts, having little previous experience of workforce planning, produced quite vague statements. In the absence of robust information, RHAs often took decisions as to how these statements were to be modified, submitted such revised information to the Department of Health and entered into educational 'contracts' on the basis of this. RHAs did make strenuous efforts to improve the quality of local workforce planning to obtain valid information, which they in turn acted upon. An example of this was *The People Pack*, produced for all NHS trusts by North East and South East Thames Regional Health Authorities (Meadows *et al.*, 1993). However, there remained the suspicion that while NHS trusts merely had to provide information to RHAs who managed the rest of the education and training process (including contracting), their interest would be limited. Indeed, Rankin and Gill (1992) argued that without involving trusts in the contracting process it was unlikely that trusts would see any incentive to improve their workforce planning approaches, through a 'lack of ownership'.

The original Working Paper 10 proposed that, over time, trusts and other NHS providers could take a greater role in the broader education and training and contracting processes. The mechanisms for this were to be via 'consortia' of local NHS employers. This was in line with the fundamental principle on which the NHS reforms of the early 1990s were based, namely that decisions should be taken at, and operational responsibility devolved to, the lowest possible levels.

Progress on the development of consortia was slow in the 1990s, with a few notable exceptions (Humphreys and Davis, 1995). The reasons for this are varied, but two key issues influenced the pace of change. Firstly, the process of developing workforce planning continued, albeit at a slow pace. Many RHAs felt uncomfortable about devolving operational responsibilities until this system was more robust. As a result significant amounts of time continued to be allocated to improving workforce planning through a mixture of training courses, manuals and development of computer models. Secondly, the early 1990s saw much time spent on relocating education and training providers from their parochial NHS homes to higher education institutions, mainly universities. Humphreys and Quinn (1994) provide a detailed explanation of the reasons behind this move, but in summary the changes in nursing education (Project 2000 – UKCC, 1986) and greater partnerships with higher education that occurred as a result, together with the anomaly of district health authorities effectively providing education services to NHS trusts from whom they also purchased health care, meant that a potential solution to a potential problem presented itself. By 1995 the majority of NHS education was provided out of higher education institutions.

The development of current consortium arrangements

The year of 1993 saw further reorganization within the NHS (Department of Health, 1994), the aim of which was to reduce bureaucracy, primarily by abolishing regional health authorities and replacing them with eight regional 'outposts' of the NHS Executive (formerly the NHS Management Executive). Given the role that RHAs had taken in education and training of the workforce, alternative arrangements had to be considered.

The arrangements for education and training were fully outlined in an NHS Executive letter (EL (95)27). The key principle of these arrangements was that education consortia were to be formalized, their membership to include NHS trusts, health authorities, primary care (GPs), social services and the independent health-care sector. The consortia were given a whole range of functions, coordinating workforce planning statements and estimating demand for staff being immediate requirements, with involvement in the contracting process developing over time. This latter responsibility was to be devolved to consortia on the basis of an assessment of their capability to manage the process, the earliest date for control over contracting (and therefore operational responsibility for budgets) being April 1996. At the same time a 'national levy' was agreed to fund such education and training and devolved in the first instance to the regional outposts of the NHS Executive, who, whatever the pace of operational devolution, would retain a strategic overview of the process and the power to alter unreasonable or poorly formulated contracting plans.

Progress to date

Consortia have spent a considerable amount of time in the past year or so in developing their internal management arrangements and understanding the contracts for which they, potentially, have responsibility. This in itself has been time-consuming, not least because of some of the complexities relating to the existing educational contracts. In order to manage the transition of education provider from the NHS to the higher education sector contracts are invariably of a long-term, 'rolling' (renewed for further periods annually) nature. This was necessary to manage some of the risks involved in taking on such large volumes of 'business'. Additionally, the consortia have created a forum where many potentially 'competing' NHS trusts and their local health authority purchaser are having to collaborate rather than compete, and where the members of the consortia need to agree 'lead' responsibilities among themselves for the range of responsibilities they have to undertake. Edmonstone (1995) has pointed out that this will be one of the many potential problem areas that will confront consortia. However, in spite of these issues some consortia have operational responsibility at this time.

Potential 'problem' areas

Edmonstone (1995), as has already been mentioned, sees a number of potential difficulties for consortia. The question of tension between members has already been considered but additional difficulties could surface in the following areas.

Workforce planning

The historical difficulties in obtaining accurate workforce planning information have already been touched on in this chapter. However, the need for common approaches among disparate members remains an important hurdle, especially since workforce planning continues to be a relatively low priority area when seen alongside the complexities of delivering cost-effective health care. The question of confidentiality is also seen as problematic if, as is sensible, workforce plans are based on the 'business planning' predictions of each NHS provider. There will also be potential conflict if one consortium member is well versed in workforce planning and sees the need for a significantly different type, or different numbers, of staff than other more 'traditional' consortia members.

The role of the NHS Executive

While the new arrangements are meant to provide for a high degree of decentralization to consortium members, the potential for NHS Executive involvement to veto proposals remains, either at Regional Office (the 'outposts') or centrally. This could occur under a number of circumstances but two in particular are realistic scenarios. Firstly, where a particular consortium has very different plans from others within the Regional Office geographical area (urban *versus* rural consortia, for example) the potential exists for the Regional Office to demand that the consortium 'plays safe'. Secondly, where validated plans come into conflict with national priorities and the political influences associated with them the Regional Office might also intervene.

Timescales

The alignment of timescales also presents a potential problem area for consortia. As already mentioned, education contracts are of a fairly long duration, typically 5 years. This period allows 1 year to negotiate contracts, 3 years for the actual education and 1 year to place and assess newly qualified staff. It also, of course, provides a sense of security for education providers. This cycle is, however, not consistent with planning horizons within the NHS. Health-care contracts are typically of 1 year's duration and this 'short-termism' can lead to instability among NHS providers. In terms of education, two problems could arise. Firstly, providers might not have the jobs to meet the supply of newly qualified staff (although opportunities might exist elsewhere); secondly, the need to make changes year on year might cause providers to require new skills over much shorter timescales than education contracts allow. This might result in providers expressing dissatisfaction with the speed of response of the education provider and creating their own 'in-house' capability for training, which may lead them to question the value of consortia.

Financial issues

A number of financial issues will place pressure on consortia. Firstly providers and the consortia are likely to incur costs in setting up the consortium processes. Central management of each consortium is required, with each typically appointing a 'project manager'. Furthermore, it is likely that if consortia members are to develop workforce planning in a robust way they will need to strengthen the function at provider level. Both of these points will result in increased transaction costs for the consortia and may not lead to savings over the original Working Paper 10 infrastructure costs.

Secondly, issues will inevitably arise around how the consortium's 'operational budget' will be used. Much of the budget will be tied up in long-term contracts; it is therefore unlikely that much of the levy will be available, certainly in the early years, to purchase a broader range or different type of training. Particular issues are likely to arise involving funding postbasic education (protected at a certain level for nurses and particular nursing courses, although perhaps a rather narrow range), management development (which was often funded separately by RHAs) and training for a wider range of staff. All of these areas are likely to be a cause of friction among consortium members.

Thirdly and finally, the very fact that large sums of money are involved in the educational contracts means that significant management time will need to be devoted to ensuring that this public money is well spent. The danger exists that financial issues will dominate consortia, and that other equally important issues such as workforce planning and demand estimation will not be given sufficient attention.

Operation of the system

Although long-term contracts exist, consortia are under no obligation to continue to purchase from local education providers. The solvency of many large educational institutions (or certainly the health science element within them) is potentially only guaranteed by a single contract with a single consortium. Edmonstone (1995) has articulated that, while survival could be an issue under this system, too much use of contractual power by consortia could result in a reduced number of education providers interested in this market, thereby increasing their relative 'power as suppliers' (Porter, 1980). The results of this could be higher costs to the NHS or a move to setting up more 'in-house' educational provision!

Consortium impact on the NHS nursing workforce

According to the IES survey (1996), education commissions in 1996/97 and 1997/98 are likely to be 14% higher than 1995/96. Thus, consortia are starting to act to redress the imbalance between the supply of and demand for nurses. However, it has already been pointed out that this is unlikely to impact on the workforce until the year 2000 at the earliest. As the survey also shows that nurses are continuing to leave the profession in significant numbers, there is no guarantee that this will redress the imbalance on its own. Indeed, the Audit Commission report (1997) would seem to suggest that core reasons for dissatisfaction at work need to be tackled if turnover and wastage are to be addressed effectively. If consortia are to genuinely improve supply and demand for nurses they will probably need to critically consider their whole approach to workforce planning.

FROM WORKFORCE OR MANPOWER PLANNING TO STRATEGIC HUMAN RESOURCE PLANNING

Although the term 'workforce planning' has been used as a more accurate description than 'manpower planning' it will be argued that the two terms represent the same philosophy and group of approaches. 'Manpower planning' first came to prominence in the 1950s and 1960s in the context of large organizations that were relatively stable bureaucracies. To these organizations with their standardized tasks and standardized jobs, 'planning' was in itself a relatively stable set of tasks concerned with accurately predicting how people would move through organizations and how many and what type would need to be recruited. In this environment manpower planning consisted of a range of activities to provide 'right' answers to the manpower needs of the organization. Typically these tasks would include the following.

- **Stocktaking**: This task was a largely numerical exercise that related to estimating the existing manpower resources of the organization. More sophisticated versions would look at recording qualitative as well as quantitative information, such as recording the skills each individual possessed. Traditionally, this process has painted a rather limited picture of the workforce and its characteristics, but this may be traced back to the stable environment and 'standardization' of the time in which the approach was developed.

- **Forecasting supply**: Understanding the internal supply within an organization was the main task of manpower planning in the 1960s; it also preoccupied much of NHS workforce planning up until the internal market reforms. A whole range of mathematical techniques were employed to allow the manpower planner to develop models to accurately forecast what was happening to the workforce and create a series of 'what if' scenarios to predict future labour turnover and stability. It is not surprising that a range of mathematical approaches have been developed, since, as Bell (1989) demonstrated, many of the early pioneers of manpower planning were to be found in the operational research departments of large organizations such as Shell, BP and the National Coal Board.
- **Forecasting demand**: This has proved over the years to be the most difficult stage within manpower planning. Traditionally, the approach was to use the 'company plan' or, in the case of the NHS, the 5-year regional plan and assume a direct, causal link between the two in order to calculate future demand for staff. This has always been characterized as a reactive process and as such has been open to accusations of only responding to the short-term tactical needs of the organization.
- **Reconciling supply and demand**: As the name of this stage suggests, manpower planning took the (limited) information available concerning the characteristics of the workforce and the internal supply and compared these with demand requirements. Typically, this would result in very specific recommendations as to the number of recruits the organization required and when, and how many promotions should be offered in a particular year.

Problems with the traditional manpower planning approach

The 1980s saw significant criticism of the traditional manpower planning approach. While some of this was related to the poor application of inherently 'sound' techniques, much criticism was also directed at the supposed predictability of the approach. Perhaps one of the most damning criticisms of the approach came from a Director of the Institute of Manpower Studies, Purkiss, who stated:

> Manpower planning has a reputation for being academic, if not tedious. It has been written about for over 20 years, every new book the definitive version. It failed in the 1960s and 1970s. It belongs to the world of calculation, computers and big bureaucracies. (Bennison and Casson, 1984, p. ix)

Unfortunately, many of the techniques and approaches criticized by Purkiss years ago underpin much of what is deemed 'good practice' by a large number of consortium members. The NHS Executive publication designed to support consortia workforce planning (NHS Executive, 1996) contains a range of forecasting techniques and methods of numerical analysis. Perhaps given the need for consortia to predict future numbers of students/newly qualified staff required this is inevitable, but it will do little to address current skill shortages, wastage and turnover rates. To properly address these areas we need to consider how 'manpower planning' has developed into the less prescriptive, less methodologically intensive approach that can be labelled 'strategic human resource planning'.

Strategic human resource planning

This is not the place to enter into the debate surrounding the term 'human resource management' (see Legge, 1995, for an excellent overview of the academic debate). The 'strategic human resource planning' approach has grown out of two series of academic developments that were well documented in the 1980s and 1990s. The first of these relates to current approaches to business strategy and business planning. Mintzberg (1994) charts how strategic planning has moved from an emphasis on a highly bureaucratic, structured process concerned with producing accurate 'right answer' corporate plans to becoming a learning process that seeks to 'reduce uncertainty' rather than produce 'magic answers'. Such a change can be characterized by the increasing use of approaches such as 'scenario planning', which seek to create internally consistent 'visions of the future' that can be utilized to think more broadly about the future direction and environment that organizations face. The second area of development has been in the personnel/human resource management debate. Human resource management is meant to represent a more strategic (aligned to the aims of the organization), more integrated approach than traditional personnel management. In terms of planning this means that greater emphasis must be placed on understanding and relating to an organization's aims and the need to ensure that planning goes beyond mere numbers to understand some of the cultural and behavioural issues involving the workforce. Rothwell (1995) argues that such a strategic human resource planning approach will not just cover the traditional supply and demand questions but will also include considerations of recruitment and retention, succession planning, career planning and labour flexibility. It is this type of comprehensive approach that is likely to offer a more coherent solution to the supply and demand imbalance that faces the NHS nursing workforce.

APPLYING A 'STRATEGIC HUMAN RESOURCE PLANNING' APPROACH TO THE NHS NURSING WORKFORCE

It has already been argued that, while traditional workforce planning techniques are necessary for the nursing workforce (in order at the very least to improve supply), they are in themselves insufficient to tackle the current imbalance between demand and supply of nursing staff. Even if the basic workforce planning skills of consortium members improve there is no guarantee that this in itself will address the high turnover and wastage rates within the nursing workforce nor the key reasons why nurses are leaving the NHS (IES, 1996). A more integrated approach is required, one that incorporates Rothwell's (1995) elements of succession/career planning, recruitment and retention and the area of labour flexibility. But how might some of these contentious issues be introduced to an already disillusioned workforce? A useful starting point is to consider why staff feel disillusioned.

Changing employer/employee relationships

Before the new range of competitive pressures that face the NHS many health service staff believe a 'golden age' of stability existed. While this is not strictly true (the 1974 reorganization and the introduction of general management in the 1980s being significant upheavals themselves), there is no doubt that many NHS staff are suffering from 'change fatigue' in the 1990s. Given that much of the pressure stems from a desire to improve the 'efficiency' of the NHS, many changes have been directly related to reducing costs and inappropriate activities within the health service. This inevitably impacts on staff, since at the most basic level of the quest for efficiency they represent up to 70% of NHS costs (Meadows *et al.*, 1993). As a result of cost pressures staff are told that organizations need to 'de-layer' or 'downsize', they are told that they need to be 'flexible', both in terms of what they do and when they do it, and they are told that traditional, well-defined career paths can no longer be guaranteed. Not surprisingly, this situation has at best disillusioned staff and at worst angered them; it is not surprising in these circumstances that nearly a quarter of the sample in the IES nursing survey (1996) cited 'job dissatisfaction' as a reason for leaving the NHS. Perhaps the only surprising feature of the situation is that managers are surprised by staff reaction! However, even in situations where, on the surface, the prospects for employees look dire, some opportunities exist and are starting to be exploited by enlightened employees in both the private sector and the NHS. These opportunities relate to what is euphemistically termed the 'new deal' (in employment).

The 'new deal'

Herriot and Pemberton (1995), describing the situation facing middle and senior managers who are subject to the vagaries of 'de-layering' and 'downsizing', discuss a range of alternative approaches to managing careers and employee expectations at a time of savage cost reduction in industry. O'Sullivan (1996) extends many of these approaches to all staff affected by such structural change at work.

The 'new deal' relates to the concept of the 'psychological contract'. While all nurses will have a written contract of employment (or should have!), there is also an implicit or 'psychological' contract that outlines the expectations both the employer and the employee have of each other and how they will behave in the workplace (Makin, Cooper and Cox, 1996). In a recent report, Holbeche (1994) highlighted many of the changes to the general world of work that reflect the experiences of NHS staff as discussed above. She argues that when such radical changes take place the 'traditional' psychological contract is no longer relevant and a new contract needs to be established. It is the establishment of this new contract that is the 'new deal' in employment relationships.

The NHS is, however, a good example of what problems can arise in relation to the establishment of this 'new deal'. O'Sullivan (1996) and Holbeche (1994) describe the traditional 'deal' or psychological contract in quite similar terms, which can be articulated as:

> if the employee is loyal, works hard and meets obligations, then the employer will provide a secure job, steady pay increases, career progression and financial security as part of a successful organization.

If uncertainty and structural change mean that this is no longer achievable, the 'new deal' can be described as:

> if the employee takes responsibility and develops appropriate skills for the organization, applies them in a way that helps the organization succeed, and behaves consistently with organizational values, then the employer will provide a challenging work environment, support for development and reward for contribution, perhaps not on a lifelong basis but with the employee more employable.

This in itself may have a high degree of legitimacy and may represent a reasonable approach. However, often, and there are many NHS examples, this 'deal' or 'change in deal' is not communicated to employees. Even worse, there are many organizations where employees do not perceive this new deal as real or realistic. For these organizations and employees an 'unbalanced' psychological contract or deal is perceived, one that O'Sullivan (1996) articulates as:

> if the employee takes responsibility and develops appropriate skills for the organization, applies them in a way that helps the organization succeed, and behaves consistently with organizational values, then the employer will provide a job if they can, gestures that they care and the same pay.

It is deals of this nature that result in job dissatisfaction, wastage and high turnover, as described in the IES survey (1996).

Some NHS organizations have successfully introduced the 'new deal' to their employees. Here professional staff are starting to seek opportunities in employment that expose them to new and 'leading edge' areas of work, which provide them with a range of development opportunities and which flexibly meet their needs. Where such an approach is observable it tends to be based on quite a new approach to managing staff: one that might be said to encompass the elements of strategic human resource planning outlined by Rothwell (1995). In particular, there is a much greater degree of integration between basic workforce planning, career planning and labour flexibility. The major dilemma is to identify the mechanisms for achieving such integration. One possible approach is to better understand the motivations of the nursing workforce.

Personal motivation – a way forward?

Understanding the personal motivation of staff has developed within the NHS as a way of managing the diversity of the workforce beyond mere equal opportunities (Gill, 1996). The argument in relation to workforce planning is that, in order to overcome issues such as job dissatisfaction and the lack of faith in the 'new deal', employers must understand what motivates their staff. Schein (1993) has made a major contribution to understanding such motivations, from research originally conducted in the 1960s and 1970s but recently updated. He argues that, as careers evolve, so individuals start to look for different things in, and want to satisfy different needs through, the career. Schein identifies a number of 'personal motivators', the one over-riding need that must be satisfied, so much so that an individual will make difficult choices to achieve it. Schein calls these motivators 'career anchors'. Through his research eight such anchors have been identified.

- **Managerial competence**: For individuals who have managerial competence as their anchor the main motivator concern is with managing people and resources. Such individuals often aim to be a generalist, and any specialist post is only considered as a way of acquiring specific experiences. Promotion prospects, responsibility and leadership are all-important to such individuals.
- **Technical/functional competence**: For individuals who have this as their anchor the main motivator is seeking to develop and maintain their specialist skills and maintain specialist knowledge in a particular area.
- **Security**: For individuals who have this as their anchor, the main motivator is the provision of a safe and reliable working environment. This can be reflected in security of tenure or a desire to remain in a specific geographical location.
- **Autonomy and independence**: For individuals who have this as their anchor, the main motivator, the existence of freedom with regard to work activities, is of paramount importance. They may wish to 'set the rules' or have relatively relaxed reporting arrangements.
- **Creativity and entrepreneurship**: For individuals who have this as their anchor, the main motivator is the ability to create new products or treatments unfettered. They are likely to want to develop their own organization or 'rules'.
- **Pure challenge**: For individuals who have this as their anchor, the need to 'win' in the face of challenges or against strong competition is the main motivator.
- **Dedication to a cause**: For individuals who have this as their anchor, the values of the organization are the main motivator. They seek to work with organizations that have similar social, religious or political beliefs to their own.
- **Lifestyle integration**: For individuals who have this as their anchor, their main motivator, the question of 'balance', is vital. The ability to sensibly manage work, family and leisure activities with no one area overwhelming others is crucial.

If employers can start to understand the career anchors of their employees it will provide valuable insights into the way they behave and act. In the NHS context at least six of these anchors are relevant (creativity and entrepreneurship and pure challenge are unlikely to be too prevalent) and a number are very important, particularly to nursing staff, as the IES 1996 survey pointed out. For example, their carer responsibilities may make the 'lifestyle integration' anchor important to some while the Audit Commission report (1997) highlighted the importance of control over work to many NHS staff.

Using personal motivations to develop 'new deals'

At present many organizations are second-guessing what employees want from the working experience, the NHS among them. As a result, a range of initiatives can be observed in NHS organizations, partly to improve motivation and partly to address areas of skill shortages. These may range from offering creche facilities and training opportunities to flexible working. The problem is that, without knowing what motivates each individual, many initiatives may not have the desired effect. Consider, for example, the offering of a fixed-term contract of employment to a nurse. For someone with a general management anchor it may be attractive if it fills a skill gap, for others it may meet their requirement for lifestyle integration. However, if the individual has a security anchor it could offer nothing but anguish! What is apparent from this example is that there are no universal solutions and there is a need to consider the workforce as heterogeneous rather than homogeneous.

NHS employers who wish to be proactive in relation to the imbalance between supply and demand for nurses are starting to respond to this diversity of motivation, especially those who can see beyond the futility of pay spirals to 'poach' staff and the limited support that increasing student supply can bring. Here we are seeing innovations in terms of attracting people from beyond their own workforce to those who may currently be outside the working population. At the same time they will be seeking to understand the motivations of their current staff and to meet these expectations. This is, however, a slow process, especially given the change fatigue felt by many in the NHS.

Clearly the NHS, as a publicly funded, politically sensitive and cash-limited service, will not be able to meet the aspirations of every single employee all of the time. However, the use of central initiatives to meet the needs of people with potentially very different motivations may make the situation even worse in that they offer costly prescriptions that may only appeal to a fraction of the workforce. Only when the employer is aware of the motivations of the employee can initiatives be sensibly planned that take account of the need for a range of 'new deals'.

The role of professional development

An understanding of personal motivation is a prerequisite of 'strategically' planning the workforce. Once understood, a range of initiatives can be developed. As has already been mentioned, it will not be possible to meet every need every time, but there are areas where the NHS has a better chance of success than others: one is the area of professional development. While it is recognized that a certain degree of professional development is mandatory (UKCC, 1990), it is clear that a number of the personal motivators will rely on the provision of effective professional development opportunities (technical/functional competence and autonomy and independence, for example). Furthermore, as 'enlightened' employers seek to meet the needs of their existing staff, they need to give consideration also to prospective employees, whether currently part of or outside the working population. A range of initiatives that have been successful have included development programmes as part of 'return to work' schemes and the creation of specific development opportunities in roles or the creation of joint posts with, for example, universities. While there is not the space here for a full discussion, such development opportunities can take a number of formats, including new roles, dedicated study, joint working and self-directed learning opportunities. A combination of these can support personal motivation at the same time as ensuring that skills are acquired to meet the demands of advancing technology within the NHS.

The NHS is well placed to take steps to improve professional development and access to it. It has an ethos of education created by the high number of professionally qualified staff. While the mechanisms may currently be fragmented between individual employers and consortia, the potential remains. Most NHS providers have access to some postbasic education for their nursing staff and it is up to them to ensure that this reflects both organizational (linked to planning) and individual (linked to personal motivation) needs.

The evidence for making such opportunities available is compelling. The IES 1996 survey spoke of 23% of nurses leaving their posts to acquire new skills; the Audit Commission report (1997) highlighted the importance of training and development as a factor in determining if an individual stayed with an organization. Elsewhere Atkinson (1989) highlighted continued training and development as a 'strategic' response to skills shortages. Furthermore, as NHS organizations seek to develop a more integrated approach to 'strategic human resource planning' they will need to provide professional development opportunities to develop career planning and succession planning.

CONCLUSION – POLICY CONSIDERATIONS FOR CONSORTIA AND INDIVIDUAL NHS EMPLOYERS

This chapter has outlined the labour market situation facing NHS employers in respect of nursing staff. This shows an imbalance between current supply of and demand for staff. Education and training consortia have started to address this issue by increasing the number of education commissions to train a further number of nurses. However, at the same time it has been argued that this is only a partial solution since survey evidence suggests that an increasing number of qualified nurses are leaving the NHS through dissatisfaction or the desire to obtain new skills (47% of the IES 1996 survey). All of this is happening while a range of factors make it likely that demand will increase further.

Current NHS workforce planning provides only a partial solution in its current format, which closely mirrors the 'traditional' approaches to 'manpower planning'. While it is right and proper that a future supply of nurses is guaranteed through education commissions an imbalance will continue as long as wastage and turnover among nursing staff remain high. A first step that education consortia could take to improve this situation would be to develop a broader interpretation of workforce planning that more closely resembles the characteristics of 'strategic human resource planning'. The danger is that workforce planning has traditionally been underdeveloped in the NHS (at local level), and without investment to improve capability it will continue to merely react to education contracting cycles without addressing wider issues. Consortia will also need to develop a series of mechanisms to allow 'investment' to be made in a wider range of postbasic education to meet the needs of the existing workforce and those nurses the NHS is seeking to encourage to return to work. This will need to be undertaken sensitively, given the contracts currently in place and the volatility that could be created by significantly restructuring a contract. Only when clear views are obtained as to what professional development is required, via a better understanding of personal motivation, can the consortia begin to engage in such dialogue.

At the same time as consortia must develop their approach there is much that local NHS employers must do individually. They must communicate clearly with employees and establish what 'psychological contract' or 'deal' is available in their current circumstances. They must be reasonable in this approach since turnover suggests that nursing staff will vote with their feet if the approach takes staff for granted. Moreover, they must make strenuous efforts to understand the personal motivations of their employees and decide to what degree they can meet them. NHS employers will need to support staff in developing their careers, within the organization wherever possible but by a planned move if personal motivations cannot be satisfied. This will require a broad interpretation of career paths and may lead to careers developing in multiple directions (Holbeche (1994) terms this 'career lattices'). Moreover, NHS employers must truly treat staff as their most valuable resource rather than just state the fact in annual reports.

REFERENCES

Atkinson, J. (1989) Four stages of adjustment to the demographic timebomb. *Personnel Management*, **Aug**.

Audit Commission (1997) *Finders, Keepers: The Management of Staff Turnover in NHS Trusts*, Audit Commission, Oxford.

Bagust, A., Burrows, J. and Oakley, J. (1992) Quality or quantity. *Health Service Journal*, **6 Aug**.

Bell, D. (1989) Why Manpower Planning is back in vogue. *Personnel Management*, **July**.

Bennison, M. and Casson, J. (1984) *The Manpower Planning Handbook*, McGraw-Hill, Maidenhead.

Conroy, M. and Stidson, M. (1988) *2001: The Black Hole – An Examination of Labour Market Trends in Relation to the NHS*, Department of Health, London.

Corby, S. (1991) When two halves make total sense. *Health Service Journal*, **18 July**.

Department of Employment (1996) *Labour Force Survey – Spring 1996*, Stationery Office, London.

Department of Health (1989a) *Working for Patients*, HMSO, London.

Department of Health (1989b) *Working for Patients: Education and Training – Working Paper 10*, HMSO, London.

Department of Health (1990) *The NHS and Community Care Act*, HMSO, London.

Department of Health (1991) *Junior Doctors – The New Deal*, HMSO, London.

Department of Health (1993) *Hospital Doctors: Training for the Future – The Report of the Working Group on Specialist Medical Training*, HMSO, London.

Department of Health (1994) *Managing the New NHS: Functions and Responsibilities in the New NHS*, HMSO, London.

Edmonstone, J. (1995) A step into the unknown? The new education and training contracting arrangements. *Health Manpower Management*, **21**(6).

Gill, P. (1996) Managing workforce diversity – a response to skill shortages. *Health Manpower Management*, **22**(6).

Government Statistical Service (1996) *Health and Personal Social Services Statistics for England 1996*, Stationery Office, London.

Greenhalgh & Co. (1994) *The Interface between Junior Doctors and Nurses*, Greenhalgh & Co., Macclesfield, Cheshire.

Herriot, P. and Pemberton, C. (1995) *New Deals: The Revolution in Managerial Careers*, John Wiley, Chichester.

Holbeche, L. (1994) *Career Development in Flatter Structures*, Roffey Park Management College, Horsham.

Humphreys, J. (1994) New models in a corporate paradigm, in *Healthcare Education: The Challenge of the Market*, (eds J. Humphreys and F. M. Quinn), Chapman & Hall, London.

Humphreys, J. and Davis, K. (1995) Quality Assurance for contracting of education: a delegated system under consortia of British National Health Service Trusts. *Journal of Advanced Nursing*, **21**, 537–543.

Humphreys, J. and Quinn, F. M. (eds) (1994) *Healthcare Education: The Challenge of the Market*, Chapman & Hall, London.

IES (1996) *In the Balance: Registered Nurse Supply and Demand, 1996*, Institute of Employment Studies, Brighton.

Legge, K. (1995) *Human Resource Management: Rhetorics and Realities*, Macmillan, Basingstoke.

Makin, P., Cooper, C. and Cox, C. (1996) *Organisations and the Psychological Contract*, British Psychological Society, Leicester.

Meadows, S. (1997) The issues surrounding the implementation of the Calman report on postgraduate training. Unpublished report on behalf of the Inner London Personnel Directors.

Meadows, S., Gill, P., Hearne, P. *et al.* (1993) *The People Pack – a Step by Step Guide to Getting the Best from Your Workforce*, Outset, Battle, Sussex.

Mintzberg, H. (1994) *The Rise and Fall of Strategic Planning*, Prentice-Hall, Hemel Hempstead.

NHS Management Executive Value for Money Unit (1990) *The Role of Nurses and Other Staff in Outpatients Departments*, HMSO, London.

NHS Executive (1995) *Education and Training in the New NHS*, NHS Executive, Leeds.

NHS Executive (1996) *Guide to Workforce Planning in Consortia*, NHS Executive, Leeds.

OPCS (1995) *Department of Health: Departmental Report 1995*, HMSO, London.

Oram, M. and Wellins, R. S. (1995) *Re-engineering's Missing Ingredient – The Human Factor*, IPD, London.

O'Sullivan, J. (1996) Managing diversity and the New Deal, in *Towers Perrin's Perspectives on Performance through People 13*, TPF&C, London.

Porter, M. (1980) *Competitive Strategy*, Free Press, New York.

Rankin, P. and Gill, P. (1992) Implementing Working Paper 10 in South East Thames: issues and options. Unpublished paper for South East Thames Regional Health Authority.

Review Body for Nursing Staff, Midwives and Professions Allied to Medicine (1996) *Thirteenth Report on Nursing Staff, Midwives and Health Visitors 1996*, Stationery Office, London.

Robinson, R. and Le Grand, J. (eds) (1994) *Evaluating the NHS Reforms*, King's Fund, London.

Rothwell, S. (1995) Human resource planning, in *Human Resource Management: A Critical Text*, (ed. J. Storey), Routledge, London.

Schein, E. H. (1993) *Career Anchors: Discovering Your Real Values*, revised edn, Pfeiffer & Co., London.

UKCC (1986) *Project 2000: A New Preparation for Practice*, UKCC, London.

UKCC (1990) *The Report of the Post-Registration Education and Practice Project*, UKCC, London.

Monitoring to keep the patient safe: an essential nursing activity

6

Maureen Theobald

I am writing this chapter with the wish that the professional issue of monitoring as a nursing activity be seen in the context of current health service delivery: the duty to the public to ensure that money is spent appropriately and to good effect; the expectation that nurse managers will provide a nursing strategy in accordance with the organization's business plan and the workforce necessary to deliver a nursing service within the planned strategy; the chief executive's duty to ensure patient safety and the risk management strategy in relation to this last issue.

The phenomenon of nursing – and nursing is properly called a phenomenon (something that appears real to the senses, regardless of whether its underlying existence is proved or its nature understood) – is claimed to be that which is expressed in and through the practice of nursing. Historians have documented well the stages of its development, through which changes have occurred. Attempts have been made to provide definitions of nursing but a review of such definitions leads one to believe that an understanding of the phenomenon is not well served by definitions.

The 29th edition (1971) of *Black's Medical Dictionary* says that professional nursing falls within four divisions: hospital nursing, private nursing, district nursing and midwifery nursing. These four categories echo the language used by Florence Nightingale in 1869 but do little to increase our understanding of the nature of nursing. 'Hospital nursing' suggests no more than where nursing might take place, whereas 'private nursing' could refer either to the nurse in her occupational capacity or to the status of the patient. 'District nursing' suggests where the nursing might take place and 'midwifery nursing' refers to the nursing that takes place in relation to a woman and childbirth. No description of practice is made, nor is mention made of the phenomenon of nursing as a legal entity; the fact that nursing accountability is written in statute and has been since 1919 finds no place in the dictionary definition.

Bertha Harmer's definition of nursing (1922) says:

> Nursing is rooted in the needs of humanity and is·founded on the ideal of service. Its object is not only to cure the sick and heal the wounded but to bring health and ease, rest, and comfort to mind and body, to shelter, nourish and practice and to minister to all those who are helpless or handicapped, young, aged or immature. Its object is to prevent disease and to preserve health. Nursing is, therefore, linked with every other social agency which strives for the prevention of disease and the preservation of health. The nurse finds herself not only concerned with the care of the individual but the health of people.

This definition refers largely to the purpose of nursing, which is a necessary as well as useful dimension to explore, whereas Virginia Henderson's definition – and it is generally accepted that Virginia Henderson's definitions of 1955 and 1966 build directly upon Harmer's – is more circumscribed and offers welcome outcome measures on the effectiveness of nursing should anyone be looking for them. Its weakness is a heavy reliance on uniqueness of functions when those identified are clearly not unique to the nurse. Had she wished to establish uniqueness then perhaps she would have done better to look to a uniqueness of purpose.

The 1966 definition says:

> The unique function of the nurse is to assist the individual, sick or well, in the performance of those activities contributing to health or its recovery (or to peaceful death) that he could perform unaided if he had the necessary strength, will or knowledge. And to do this in such a way as to help him gain independence as rapidly as possible.

.This definition concentrates on broad functions that clearly are not unique to the nurse, although it perhaps expresses what could be claimed by the nurse as nursing and what the profession of nursing, other health-care professionals, society at large and political will **could** make unique to nursing should such bodies so choose. It is also appropriate to remember that both Henderson and Harmer were born in the last century and experienced nursing in the early part of this one. They were greatly concerned to distinguish nursing from non-nursing in their fight to gain professional recognition of nursing, and their definitions reflect this.

Hildegard Peplau (1952) stated that 'Human relationship between an individual who is sick, or in need of health services, and a nurse especially educated to recognise and to respond to the need for help' defines nursing. Yet it clearly does not, in that the words used are insufficient to do so. To suggest that nursing exists because there is a nurse involved might be the case in a limited use of the language, but is not helpful to any further understanding.

The first edition of the *Reader's Digest Universal Dictionary* (1986) does not consider nursing at all, even though it goes to great lengths to explain the use of the word 'nurse'. An assumption, perhaps, as with Peplau (1952), that nursing is what nurses do. And, bearing in mind that to seek an understanding of the phenomenon of nursing through a dictionary definition or, indeed, anyone else's definition is to court certain disappointment, 'nursing is what nurses do' is not necessarily as unhelpful as it might first appear. I suggest this not least because it can encourage us to look away from definitions and further towards an exploration of the phenomenon of nursing. And this approach is favoured because phenomena require description rather than definition and this in itself insists that we look closely at what is there and try to gain an understanding.

Progress is made by Josephine E. Paterson and Loretta T. Zderad in *Humanistic Nursing* in their consideration of a phenomenological approach to nursing. A summarized description is given by Praeger and Hogarth, in George (1985), where the stages stated in such an approach are as follows.

1. **Preparation of the nurse knower for coming to know**. This stage includes a thorough study of the humanities for the understanding of the nature of being, together with an acknowledged value of the experience of an individual.
2. **Nurse knowing the other intuitively**. This stage refers to getting inside the other person's experience sufficiently well to merge the self with the rhythmic spirit of the other.
3. **Nurse knowing the other scientifically**. This stage requires analysis of that which is considered to be known intuitively in order to sort out and categorize it.
4. **Nurse complementarily synthesizing known others**. This stage requires the taking into account of the experiences and knowledge of other nurses, with the suggested outcome of grasping a principle.
5. **Succession within the nurse from the many to the paradoxical one**. This last phase contains the articulated vision of experience and looks to compare favourably with Schon's reflective practice theory.

The strength of Paterson and Zderad's approach lies in the recognition of the practice element in the production of theory. 'Theory development begins with description', Praegar and Hogarth state (ch.16, p. 293). Paterson and Zderad do not attempt to find a model and apply it to a nursing situation, as did some nurse theorists who invented models of nursing in the 1960s and 1970s. And they introduce the issue of the nature of nursing knowledge. They do demonstrate a weakness, however, which lies in the taking of too much for granted; a too heavy reliance upon unexplained assumptions. And some argue, with justification, that the language they use is not welcoming to those who have not studied in this area.

This author believes, however (Theobald, 1984), that a nurse in practice learns that s/he may find him/herself in situations in which s/he must demonstrate that s/he is prepared to listen even to those who indicate that they would rather not have to talk, such as may occur with patients suffering from a mental health problem, and s/he must be ready to talk to those who sometimes choose not to listen, such as those persons who demonstrate anger and abuse in an accident and emergency department. S/he must learn to show empathy through body movements and facial expression, for not all patients will have good hearing, and must learn what physical proximity might mean to all, especially to those patients from ethnic minorities whose culture may be less familiar, in order to avoid offence or embarrassment. It is necessary for the nurse to come to terms with the ultimate inevitability of his/her own future death in order to be able to help those persons who may be approaching theirs. S/he must learn what it means to be a professional person, and accept the responsibility of accountability. And s/he will have to decide how this person who accepts such accountability differs from the person s/he may have considered him/herself to be before. The nurse's practice skills must be based upon an accepted body of knowledge, as to work with less might hinder the patient's recovery or place the patient in danger. The nurse must learn how to offer help without imposing his/her will upon another person; this may sometimes involve helping persons see for themselves their new limitations which have resulted from injury or disease process and enabling them to grow towards an acceptance of them. This may involve the nurse in offering him/herself as either a mental, emotional or physical support, until the sick person grows able to cope without such support or else learns to supply their own. And this contains a tacit consent to the patient being an autonomous person, one who sees him/herself as free to exercise the right to self-direction (Theobald, 1984).

Nursing is generally considered to be a practice-based discipline and for my purpose I am prepared to take this as a given, even though the term 'practice' is used differently by individual non-nurses and also differently by individual nurses. Language has many attributes, one of which must be the ability to illuminate rather than to obscure if, like truth, it helps us make sense of our world. This lack of clarity concerning essential words on the part of nurses serves to confuse further our general usage of many terms. The need we have to describe nursing in an understandable way is impeded if the very words we use have no common meaning and may be interpreted differently by individual nurses.

Nursing is what nurses practise, and such practice is whatever they are duty bound to do in the interest of their patients during their shift or work period. It concerns whatever the nurse involves him/herself in after s/he has said 'on duty'.

Nursing issues may be considered within the dimensions of clinical practice, management, teaching and research, but nursing practice is the central discipline upon which management, teaching and research in nursing depend. Nursing management does not exist outside nursing practice and the same may be said of nursing education (teaching) and nursing research. The author is aware of the tendency, or at least the potential, for the practice of either management, teaching or research to distort the practice of nursing as well as to contribute to it, but this potential cannot be explored here and it is neither beneficial nor necessary to this chapter to do so. For the purpose of exploring the nature of nursing, only clinical practice will be considered and hopefully in this way the potential for distortion will be removed.

Clinical practice itself, however, may also be categorized in a variety of ways, according to the purpose of the categorization, for nursing activities can be broadly identified as interventions and treatments, communications and monitoring. Further categorization of nursing activities may be considered, into activities of daily living, occupation-specific duties, non-invasive clinical treatments, invasive clinical treatments, communications and monitoring. It is neither possible nor intentional to refer further to any activities other than monitoring within this chapter.

And it can be argued that nursing practice requires knowledge for what to do and knowledge for how to do it, knowledge for determining whether to do it at all, which requires knowledge for an understanding, and knowledge for whether it should be done by oneself or by another. There is knowledge that is needed so as to determine how to act, which also incorporates, although it is different from, whether to act at all. And whether to act will be determined by the quality of understanding of the issues involved and the ability to discriminate between the normal and the abnormal. But examples are needed in order to make sense of these statements, and they will be provided.

Eraut (1994) considers knowledge creation and knowledge use in professional contexts, and although he does not specifically address the nursing issue there are parallels to be drawn regarding professional knowledge that are useful to consider. He suggests that there are traditional assumptions about both the labelling and packaging of knowledge that need to be challenged. This is surely true of nursing knowledge, which is so frequently treated as though there is only one kind, and possibly trivialized as a result.

As Schon (1985) says:

> It is difficult for [professionals] to imagine how to describe and teach what might be meant by making sense of uncertainty, performing artistically, setting problems, and choosing among competing professional paradigms, when these processes seem mysterious in the light of the prevailing model of professional knowledge.

Thus, in order to consider monitoring appropriately in this wider context, monitoring itself also requires to be seen within a knowledge context, if we are to understand just what sort of activity it is and perhaps to hold a view of the nature of the knowledge required in its practice. It is evident that if we acknowledge the complexities of nursing practice much of what we understand nursing practice to be cannot be observed. And if we look at the words 'function' and 'purpose' more closely, the issue of the non-observable in nursing might be more clearly understood.

Functions can be expressed in action or performance and are intended to serve or achieve a particular purpose or purposes. For example, the action of winding a clock relates to the function of the key, which is to wind the clock with the purpose of setting the clock to work. It is not necessary to know how to build a clock in order to wind it efficiently and without causing harm. But neither is it sufficient simply to know how to achieve the physical act of winding with the key. Damage to the clock can occur and should be prevented. For the person winding the clock needs to know how to recognize the resistance against the winding action that is noticed when the clock's mechanism is nearing the position of being fully wound or else overwinding can occur and the clock's spring can be broken. This knowledge is not observable in the action of winding the clock. Or consider the action of placing a thermometer under a patient's tongue in relation to the function of the thermometer to register a temperature, which in turn will serve the purpose of finding out the patient's body temperature. It is not necessary to know how the thermometer is constructed in order to use it properly, nor is it necessary to have an understanding of what the human body temperature normally is in order to record a person's body temperature. But it is necessary to know what a normal body temperature is for the recording to have any meaning to the recorder. Function concerns itself with what and how and is potentially visible, whereas purpose concerns itself with the reason why and is more likely to be invisible.

Nursing and the nurse's role are frequently described in terms of functions, by which I mean that observers concern themselves with identifying exactly what nurses can be seen to do – what actions they take – in the course of a shift, a span of duty, management of a patient caseload or a particular intervention, in order to state what nursing and the nurse's role are. These observable functions are argued to be what comprises the role of the nurse and as such offer professional parameters. I would wish to argue that role, as identified through observable functions alone, is an inadequate determinant of nursing borders. For when a nurse functions, acts or performs, she is engaged in nursing practice, only some of which is observable. Nursing practice, however, encompasses the unobservable also, as in the example of clock-winding or temperature-taking, and this latter is concerned more with purpose or reasons why. Another example of this phenomenon is the clinical decision-making required of an individual practitioner that is referred to by Benner (1984), such as when a nurse decides to inspect a wound site on the basis that the body temperature is raised above normal some days after surgery when there is no visible sign of a chest infection or urinary tract infection. The nurse does this because s/he knows that a raised temperature in a postoperative patient is one possible sign of wound infection.

I wish to explore the issue of monitoring, firstly because of its importance as a nursing activity and secondly because, although arguably central to the purpose of nursing, I consider it to be an issue that is very much neglected when attempts are made to clarify nursing practice and the knowledge required to ensure safe practice. Nurses, such as Henderson (1966) and Wright (1986) who wish to develop the professional status of nursing have chosen to seek an exclusive role for nurses. This has proved very difficult to achieve, and I believe such a quest to be less than helpful in serving the best interests of patients. Yet the activity of monitoring is undoubtedly special, so please join me in an exploration of the concept of monitoring in order to achieve clarity in at least this one aspect of nursing practice.

The word 'monitoring' suggests watchfulness or a mindful observation of a thing or a person, from the Latin *monere*, 'to warn'. In some contexts, such as in the classroom, monitoring is performed by a person who is called a monitor and is usually a pupil. In this case the monitor might be an aid to the teacher, as in the example of a classroom register monitor who is required to inform the teacher of absent pupils. Such a monitor might also be used to observe and report on the behaviour of other children and then to admonish or caution those other children as a result of the monitoring activity or to inform a teacher so that admonishment or caution is carried out. In these instances the monitor is a person and the monitoring is either of other persons or of written records concerning the activities of other persons.

But a monitor is not always a person, although it might be an aid to someone who has the responsibility to monitor. The word 'monitor' is also used to describe a piece of apparatus such as a television set, which shows images for transmission, as in the closed-circuit television used in security systems. Or the information-gathering aspect of monitoring might be achieved through the data display on a computer. In this extended use of the word the monitor is an instrument through which information for the purpose of monitoring is obtained.

So it seems clear even from this brief exposition that monitoring involves the exercise of observation in order to gain information that, once gained, will need to be interpreted in order to be understood. Following interpretation, which results in the meaning of the information gathered becoming clear, and the relevance of the information in a given situation being known and understood, a decision concerning possible action will be enabled.

In the context of health-care delivery, particularly within an acute hospital setting, patients are monitored for a variety of reasons and in a variety of ways, some of which we will explore. Yet it remains the case that the exercise of monitoring is performed in order to gain information that will ultimately lead to the possibility of action being taken. In nursing it is the nurse who is the monitor, the recorder of information; the nurse who has the responsibility for monitoring. This is an occupational duty that has implications for the nurse in relation to her recorded status on the national register as well as for the risk management strategy of the organization that employs her. These two issues will be discussed at length later.

To say that the nurse has the responsibility for monitoring is not the same as saying that only nurses are able to perform the monitoring function, but rather that, because nurses are the members of the health-care team with a 24-hour presence and a 24-hour responsibility for continuity of care (following the acceptance of the clinical grading criteria for nurses, midwives and health visitors introduced in 1987), the responsibility of overall monitoring is expected of them, and they are accountable for its maintenance.

Nurses are not alone in the act of monitoring. There is no denying that doctors monitor the effect of their interventions or treatments. A surgeon, for example, does not perform an operation upon a patient and then walk away without a backward glance. S/he visits the patient once returned from the theatre to the ward and then after discharge through an outpatient clinic or a GP practice. And a physician monitors the therapeutic and side-effects of medical treatment s/he has prescribed, whether directly or through a nursing report. Similarly physiotherapists and occupational therapists monitor the effect of their treatments. The same can be said of all health-care workers in relation to the contribution they make to the treatment or care that a patient receives, because it falls within the expectations of professional obligation. In this way nurses are no different from other health-care professionals, in that they share a similar obligation to monitor the effects of their own interventions.

But the nurse's overarching monitoring duty is not just in relation to her own interventions. The function of patient monitoring as a different activity for the nurse – one over and above that expected of other health-care workers – is to serve the specific purpose of keeping the patient safe: a 24-hour responsibility. For safety is the minimum that patients and their relatives expect from any health services they might receive and it is the minimum duty that a nurse owes to her patients. This concept is one that is included in Florence Nightingale's standard 'that the hospital should do the patient no harm'. And this is one of the ways in which nurses form a part of the armoury within the organization's risk management strategy, because in employing a nurse the employers know that they have the right to expect that patients within the charge of the nurse will be kept safely.

For although the surgical operation might be successful from the surgeon's point of view, it requires the monitoring vigilance of the nurse in the postoperative period for that success to be maintained. And, similarly, the physiotherapist might be satisfied that the patient can walk unaided during the day, but s/he knows that it requires the vigilance of the nurse to monitor the patient when s/he gets up during the night. And though the dietitian can determine the most balanced diet, yet the nurse is required to monitor what the patient eats, together with any following effect. And this monitoring of a patient and the effects of the interventions of other health-care workers upon him or her is now an integral part, in that it cannot be separated from the rest of what is understood to be nursing practice.

The mindful observation contained in the action of monitoring is a skill essential to nursing that is practised by nurses in all the branches of nursing – adult, sick children, mental health and mental handicap. It is a skill that must be learned; one that requires knowledge in order to practise competently – which in turn requires opportunities for practice in order to develop the necessary expertise. So what is required for the development of this skill of mindful observation?

The nurse must be aware that such observation is a nursing activity. This is part of the mindset – the learning schema – involved in becoming a nurse. The nurse must learn that, in order to monitor a patient in any context, an assessment of the patient and the situation must be made. And in order to make an assessment the nurse must learn how to assess, which in turn requires that s/he is able to make accurate observations. In order that the observations be accurate the nurse must learn exactly what must be observed. For example, the instruction 'Observe Mrs Jones' cannot reasonably be expected to deliver information on Mrs Jones other than that Mrs Jones remains in the same place – or not – as she was when the observation of her was requested. For greater detail to be delivered a closer request must be made, e.g. 'Observe Mrs Jones's skin'. But even this will not suffice, for if such an instruction is given to an individual that individual will have to decide for him/herself whether to observe the colour, the temperature to touch or the visual health (e.g. with or without spots or other markings or the wholeness of it). Therefore it matters – even if for no other reason than an efficient use of time – that, for appropriate observations to be made, the context in which they are to be made is known by the observer. What might sensibly be considered as an efficient use of time in this context, however, is the opportunity to develop the necessary skilled competence and expertise; that skilled competence and expertise expected of the skilled nurse.

And when one refers to a skilled nurse or an expert nurse, the language used often refers to an experienced nurse – language that needs to be unpacked in order to appreciate fully what might be contained within it. For an experience or a number of experiences are required in order to become experienced in anything, yet the nature of experience can be misunderstood.

The nature of experience as an entity suggests more than simply an event that has occurred. For example, the passing of a car may be described as an event, but as an event it might pass unnoticed. As such it cannot be claimed as an experience by an individual who did not notice it. For the passing of a car to become an experience for an individual it has to be noted by that individual. The taking of such notice, which changes the passing of the car from an event into an individual experience, does not assume any understanding by the individual. For example, the experience of a passing car may be obtained by an individual who lives in an underdeveloped country and who has never seen or heard of a car before. Nevertheless, the reality of the experience as an experience is not changed by such a lack of understanding, because the individual – given a normal intelligence and language skills – will be able to recount the experience in a way that makes it recognizable to someone who has any such understanding, i.e. is able to recognize the description of a passing car. Therefore it may be said that an experience is an occurrence that has significance to the recipient of the experience but is not necessarily fully understood by him/her. But it is not suggested that the phrase 'an experienced nurse' is intended to mean a nurse who has gained experience but who has little understanding of the experience gained. So it matters to our enquiry to determine why this is the case.

We have seen that it can be argued that gaining experience is no more than the acquisition of a number of noticed events. Such events may be of the same category, as in noting the repeated events of passing cars. The cars would not have to be the same either in design, size or colour, for example, for the individual to claim to have experienced the passing by of many cars. Such experience would enable the individual to cease to be surprised by the event and might reach a point where the experience was so familiar that the event of a passing car went unnoticed. But for such an event to move from event to experience and back again to event a change must occur in the perception of the event of the passing car by the individual, by which I mean that for the passing car to be ignored by the individual for whom it was once an experience, an understanding of what the passing car now represents to him/her must have been gained. For the individual no longer to be surprised or frightened or excited or pleased or angered or threatened by the passing car s/he must have gained an understanding of what a passing car means to him/her in the context in which s/he finds him/herself. Had any of these changes not come about the individual would have continued to notice the event of the passing car. Every passing car would continue to be an event. In order to identify the reasons why the changes occurred empirical studies are required that are not within the scope of this work, but whatever the cause of the change it is undeniable that some change took place.

In nursing, the expression 'gaining experience' refers to the opportunity to be in patient-related situations and to learn from those situations. Nurses are expected to gain experience **of** X in order to become experienced **in** X.

To become experienced, therefore, a nurse requires to be exposed to the event in which experience is to be gained, and with repeated opportunities to identify and assess similar bodies of information in recognizable contexts. And in order to make room for the many experiences s/he must acquire in order to become experienced in all of them the nurse needs the opportunity for exposure to events so that the noticed events may become experiences. Thus s/he will be an experienced nurse for whom the experiences not only have meaning but are those of which s/he has an understanding. This does, of course, have implications for anyone organizing nursing service delivery and for those involved in planning learning opportunities for student nurses. The nurse when monitoring can only monitor safely when s/he is experienced in that which s/he is required to monitor and on which s/he might be required to act.

It remains to be said, however, that, although monitoring requires an experienced nurse and the overall aim of monitoring is to keep the patient safe, not all monitoring activities can be categorized in the same way. This fact in turn requires some attention if we are to make use of our understanding of the monitoring function and the implications of some current nursing skills mix patterns. The following are examples of monitoring activities that may be undertaken by nurses.

In nursing, some activities that can be called monitoring activities involve the monitoring of treatments and their efficacy as well as the patient's reactions to them. An example of this type of monitoring activity is found in the monitoring of a patient receiving an intravenous infusion. It can be readily seen that this combination of the monitoring activity with a therapeutic intervention requires close observation of both the patient and the equipment to ensure that the treatment progresses according to plan. Consideration must be given to what a nurse needs to know apart from acknowledging this as a proper nursing activity, in order to determine how best it may be learned. The nurse will know that an intravenous infusion is prescribed to run through in a given time. S/he will be aware that the calculation of drops per minute must be correct for the infusion to run through in the desired time. S/he will know how to perform this calculation. S/he will know the complications that may occur if the infusion runs through too quickly, together with the signs of the possible complications when an infusion runs through too quickly. S/he will understand what the signs mean and who should be called in such an event. S/he will know that the infusion needle might become displaced, and what the signs of a displaced needle are. S/he will know what action to take. S/he will know that a doctor or a nurse might be asked to resite the drip. S/he will understand that the drip must be closed off if the signs of needle displacement are evident. S/he will note this on the fluid balance chart. S/he will know that an infusion may prove very uncomfortable for the patient and cause the patient to remain more immobile than is good for him/her. S/he knows that ambulation might need to be encouraged.

Monitoring the state of a patient who is attached to a cardiac monitor is an example of monitoring that involves observation of the patient as well as the equipment, although there is no direct treatment involved from the monitor. When a cardiac monitor is attached to a patient the nurse must monitor the information received through the cardiac monitor as well as monitoring the patient for signs of distress or discomfort that could result from the apparatus itself. The nurse must know that a cardiac monitor is a piece of electrical equipment that will support him/her in monitoring the state of the patient. S/he must know how to set it up and must learn how to read the cardiac tracing. S/he must know how to interpret the cardiac tracing. S/he also learns to observe the patient as well as the monitor and that a straight line tracing might mean that a wire has become disconnected. S/he must know how to report the results of the monitor, how to recognize potentially dangerous recordings and how to act in emergency situations. S/he must be mindful to care for the patient rather than the monitor. The nurse must also learn how anxious patients and relatives will be when cardiac monitoring is necessary. S/he needs to know how to empathize and comfort in order to relieve their distress.

The safe-keeping of patients may be readily understood in the activities described above, but there are other less obvious ways of monitoring when doing one's duty in keeping patients safe. An example of this is in monitoring the state of a patient's fluid balance through information gained from the data recorded on fluid charts, which requires the recording of fluid intake and output amounts accurately, and noting the difference between them. This monitoring activity is also designed to keep patients safe, but the absence of technical equipment not only removes an obvious inducement to anxiety for the patient but may also reduce the awareness of observers of any activity taking place at all. (It is also an example of an activity that requires more than observation of the activity by a non-nurse in order to deduce its purpose.) The nurse must know that fluid charts exist, together with their purpose. S/he must be aware of the relevance of maintaining a fluid chart in relation to the specific patient. S/he must know what can be recorded and where (i.e. how and where to record the amount taken in and the amount put out). S/he must understand the significance of the figures recorded and learn how to recognize important and relevant information. S/he must learn what action to take when significant information is received and recognized as such (e.g. what to do and who to inform).

Although record-keeping may not seem an obvious way of safeguarding patients, the assessing, noting and recording of the condition and progress of patients is an activity designed to achieve this purpose. And record-keeping as a monitoring activity can be extended to ensuring that care plans are up to date and will involve the nurse in knowing where to locate the care plan. The nurse will know that the vital signs are of respiration, temperature, pulse and blood pressure, and that they are to be measured and recorded, and s/he will make a decision concerning who has the knowledge and ability to do so.

A further and undramatic but no less important instance of monitoring is contained within the nurse's duty to ensure that special diets are given where appropriate. The nurse must be aware of the importance of diet in a patient's treatment and such knowledge must incorporate not only the positive effects that diet may have but also the harmful effects. This in turn requires him/her to know the condition from which the patient suffers and how to recognize benefit or harm being done to the patient according to the disease and the prognosis. And it requires that s/he builds a good and trusting relationship with the patient through skilful communication so that the patient will inform the nurse of changes in the way s/he is feeling, thus enabling the nurse to interpret and understand the changes. For action might be required in order to ensure safety.

Monitoring of the patient's spiritual safety is also the responsibility of the nurse and it is his/her duty to check the patient's religious requirements in order to avoid spiritual harm and thereby meet the patient's needs. In this way the nurse is acknowledging the patient's right to have his/her views respected whether they are shared by the nurse or not. This requires a certain maturity on the part of the nurse, who must have achieved sufficient self-awareness to understand that his/her own attitude to spirituality – whether based upon accepted religious beliefs or not – needs to be recognized. In this way s/he can feel comfortable with a patient's religion or absence of it and seek only to act in the patient's best interest. The nurse's agreement or approval of the patient's beliefs are irrelevant in this respect, because his/her duty is to keep the patient culturally safe. The nurse must know what religion the patient has and that it may matter particularly at the time of death. S/he should know of any special requirements concerning religious practice at the time of death or how to access an appropriate minister of religion. S/he must ensure that the patient's wishes are respected, and be aware that friends and relatives will be especially sensitive to details at such a time. S/he should know that the information required will be in the patient's care plan and medical notes.

The subject of practice-based knowledge is too vast to deal with in this chapter other than through a brief excursion, but it cannot be ignored entirely because of the inter-relationship of nursing practice and the knowledge required for it. The examples above indicate that a nurse needs knowledge for what to do, as well as knowledge of how to do it. S/he needs knowledge for determining whether to do it at all, which requires knowledge for an understanding in order to determine whether it should be done by oneself or by another.

Knowledge for how to do it is the practical type of knowledge expressed well by Oakeshott (1967) and is commonly thought of as know-how. Schon (1991) relabels this 'knowing-in-action'. Oakeshott distinguishes between technical and practical knowledge, considering technical knowledge to be capable of written codification and practical knowledge to be expressed only through practice. Challenges to Oakeshott's view are growing, however, which perhaps suggests that his own inability to codify was mistaken for an inability for such knowledge to be codified. Eraut (1985) claims that '[p]ractical knowledge is never tidy, an appropriate language for handling much of it has yet to be developed'. And Benner's (1984) work in exploring clinical decision-making as the core of expert nursing practice has thrown light on the knowledge creation issue. In Meerabeau's (1992) review of the various writers on the subject of expert, tacit knowledge, she examined the implications of what she terms expert knowledge for nursing research. I acknowledge her paper as a useful literary source for this subject area. Her comments on Broudy and his four distinguished modes of how knowledge is used – replication, application, interpretation and association – suggested that she and others were capable of making value judgements on the worth of the ways in which knowledge is used. This may be valid, of course, but to suggest that certain ways in which we use knowledge are somehow better than others is also open to criticism. Whereas it seems both right and proper to question the efficiency of using any method and perhaps to seek where necessary to improve the efficiency, this is quite different, I believe, from the suggestion that manners of using knowledge should be value laden and find a place in some hierarchy of worth. Meerabeau's reminder that:

> [t]he nursing profession has tended to devalue particularistic, craft-based knowledge in favour of the more generalizable, discipline-based knowledge, and it is important that enthusiasm for new nursing curricula based on Project 2000 recommendations do not over-accentuate this trend

is certainly worth noting. Within the context of the modern health service and the need to ensure that service contracts are delivered at the keenest prices, the cost of the nursing service must be assuredly value for money. In order to retain a competitive edge service managers must seek to contain staff costs and ensure that funded nursing establishments are kept to the minimum necessary to ensure quality and safety in nursing care delivery. Such actions are, of course, laudable, and I do not seek here to justify extravagant use of public monies. But within this context of value for money, employers who seek to avoid relying solely upon professional judgement to determine the number of nursing staff required per shift may choose to measure workload in order to determine a funded staffing establishment. It is not the intention to consider the varying methods of workload measurement here or their relative efficiency, but rather to highlight the fact that, bearing in mind the argument that led to the above conclusion, any workload measurement operator will obtain an incomplete measurement if they take into account only that nursing practice which is observable.

These findings also suggest that particular consideration should be given by teachers who plan clinical placement opportunities for students of nursing, because curriculum planners with the responsibility for interpreting the statutory body guidelines may place a student of nursing in a ward or department in order that they should observe nursing practice. Such a placement would be intended to benefit the student by offering the opportunity to understand nursing. Yet, as has been argued previously, the awareness that observation will enable only part of the practice of nursing to be seen should lead educators to greater realism in relation to what can be expected of a student's learning where interaction is limited or denied. The need for the student to ask questions and have them answered was demonstrated by Eraut *et al.* (1995), and the need to understand those aspects of nursing that cannot be seen has implications both for the way in which wards and departments labelled as training wards should be staffed and for the way in which education contracts are funded. For to drive down the service contract price, with a resulting reduction in the number of qualified nursing posts, will not enable the interactive learning that will prove efficient unless the education contract price reflects the essential nature of learning a practice-based discipline and includes payment for the time necessary for the nurse teacher to support the necessary interactive learning during clinical placements. These proposals in support of interactive learning relate well to the language of reflective practice, espoused in curriculum language, which encourages communication between the observer and the observed.

Monitoring, as a nursing activity designed to keep the patient safe, deserves greater attention not only from nurses themselves but also from those who employ them.

REFERENCES

Benner, P. (1984) *From Novice to Expert*, Addison-Wesley, Menlo Park, CA.

Eraut, M. (1985) Knowledge creation and knowledge use in professional contexts. *Studies in Higher Education*, **10**(2).

Eraut, M. (1994) *Developing Professional Knowledge and Competence*, Falmer Press, London

Eraut, M., Alderton, J., Boylan, A. and Wraight, A. (1995) *Learning to Use Scientific Knowledge in Nursing and Midwifery Education*, English National Board for Nursing, Midwifery and Health Visiting, London.

George, J. B., Belcher, A., Bennet, A. *et al.* (1985) *Nursing Theories*, Prentice-Hall, Englewood Cliffs, NJ.

Meerabeau, L. (1992) Tacit nursing knowledge: an untapped resource or a methodological headache. *Journal of Advanced Nursing*, **17**(1), 108–112.

Oakeshott, M. (1967) *The Concept of Education*, Routledge & Kegan Paul, London.

Schon, D. A. (1991) *The Reflective Practitioner*, Ashgate Publishing, Arena.

FURTHER READING

Alexander, M. F. (1983) *Learning to Nurse*, Churchill Livingstone, Edinburgh.

Appleton, C. (1993) The art of nursing: the experience of patients and nurses. *Journal of Advanced Nursing*, **18**(6), 892–899.

Ayer, A. J. (1971) *Language, Truth and Logic*, Penguin Books, Harmondsworth.

Ayer, A. J. (1988) *The Problem of Knowledge*, Penguin Books, Harmondsworth.

Beck, C. T. (1994) Phenomenology: its use in nursing research. *International Journal of Nursing Studies*, **31**(6), 499–510.

Behr, R. and Nolan, M. (1995) Sources of knowledge in nursing. *British Journal of Nursing*, **4**(3), 141–142, 159.

Boud, D., Keogh, R. and Walker, D (1985) *Reflection: Turning Experience into Learning*, Kogan Page, London.

Burnard, P. (1987) Towards an epistemological basis for experiential learning in nurse education. *Journal of Advanced Nursing*, **12**, 189–193.

Cahill, J. (1994) Is this the best intervention? *Professional Nurse*, **Mar.**, 394–398.

Carnevali, D. L. *et al.* (1984) *Diagnostic Reasoning in Nursing*. J. B. Lippincott, Philadelphia, PA.

Chandler, J. (1991) Reforming nurse education 1: The reorganisation of nursing knowledge. *Nurse Education Today*, **11**(1), 83–88.

Clarke, M. (1986) Action and reflection: practice and theory in nursing. *Journal of Advanced Nursing*, **11**, 3–11.

Cushing, A. (1994) Historical and epistemological perspectives on research and nursing. *Journal of Advanced Nursing*, **20**(3), 406–411.

Drummond, M. and Maynard, A. (1993) *Purchasing and Providing Cost-Effective Health Care*, Churchill Livingstone, Edinburgh.

Faulkner, A. (1985) *Nursing – A Creative Approach*, Baillière Tindall, Eastbourne.

Fradd, E. (1994) A broader scope to practice: professional development in paediatric nursing. *Child Health*, **Apr/May**, 233–238.

Goldie, S.M. (1987) *Florence Nightingale in the Crimean War 1854–56*, Manchester University Press, Manchester.

Harvey, S. (1993) The genesis of a phenomenological approach to advanced nursing practice. *Journal of Advanced Nursing*, **18**(4), 526–530.

Lacey, D. G. (1993) Discovering theory from psychiatric nursing practice. *British Journal of Nursing*, **2**(15), 763–764, 766.

Lathlean, J. (1995) *The Implementation and Development of Lecturer Practitioner Roles in Nursing*, Ashdale Press, Oxford.

Macleod, M. (1994) It's the little things that count: the hidden complexity of everyday clinical nursing practice. *Journal of Clinical Nursing*, **3**(6), 361–368

Paul, R. W. and Heaslip, P. (1995) Critical thinking and intuitive nursing practice. *Journal of Advanced Nursing*, **22**(1), 40–47.

Pearson, A. (1983) *The Clinical Nurse Unit*, Heinemann Medical Books, London.

Peters, R. S. (1970) *Ethics and Education*, Unwin University Books, London.

Pownall, M. (1991) Dual duty. *Nursing Times*, **87**(2), 21.

Taylor, B. (1993) Phenomenology: one way to understand nursing practice. *International Journal of Nursing Studies*, **30**(2), 171–179.

UKCC (1989) *Exercising Accountability: A Framework to Assist Nurses, Midwives and Health Visitors to Consider Ethical Aspects of Professional Practice*, United Kingdom Central Council for Nursing, Midwifery and Health Visiting, London.

UKCC (1992) *A Guide for Students of Nursing and Midwifery*, United Kingdom Central Council for Nursing, Midwifery and Health Visiting, London.

UKCC (1992) *Code of Professional Conduct*, United Kingdom Central Council for Nursing, Midwifery and Health Visiting, London.

UKCC (1992) *Standards for Records and Record Keeping*, United Kingdom Central Council for Nursing, Midwifery and Health Visiting, London.

UKCC (1992) *Standards for the Administration of Medicines*, United Kingdom Central Council for Nursing, Midwifery and Health Visiting, London.

UKCC (1992) *The Scope of Professional Practice*, United Kingdom Central Council for Nursing, Midwifery and Health Visiting, London.

Van der Peet, R. (1995) *The Nightingale Model of Nursing*, Campion Press.

Wright, S. (1986) *Building and Using a Model of Nursing*, Edward Arnold, London.

Wright, S. and Caulfield, H. (1994) Defining nurses' and doctors' duty of care. *Nursing Standard*, **9**(12–14), 31–32.

Young, A. (1991) *Law and Professional Conduct in Nursing*, Scutari Press, London.

7

Reflection and reflective practice

Francis M. Quinn

INTRODUCTION

Although reflection as a concept had been established in education since the turn of the century, it was the work of Donald Schon (Schon, 1983, 1987) in the mid-1980s that put it well and truly on the agenda of professional practice in both the teaching and the nursing professions. The significance of reflection in nursing lies in its close relationship to learning in professional practice settings; experiential learning is learning that results from experience and is essentially learning by doing, rather than by listening to other people or reading about it. Reflection is seen as an important component of experiential learning because it constitutes a means of thinking about professional practice.

WHAT IS MEANT BY 'REFLECTION'?

The term 'reflection' is used in a variety of ways in the literature, so it may be helpful to start from first principles in seeking to pin the concept down. Figure 7.1 gives a range of meanings of the terms 'reflect' and 'reflection', and it can be seen that reflection is a psychological construct that is closely related to a range of other internal mental (cognitive) processes such as thinking, reasoning, considering and deliberating (Gregory, 1987).

Any discussion of reflection needs to take into account a number of general assumptions about the mental processes of human beings. Since earliest times the ability to reason has been seen by philosophers as the key characteristic that distinguishes human beings from other animals, and refers to the capability of human beings for rational problem-solving and truth-seeking. This capability resides in the human mind, and some philosophers postulate a distinction between the

A. **Reflect** (from Latin *reflectere*: to bend back)
  • To consider
  • To think quietly and calmly
  • To cogitate
  • To come to remember or realize
  • To express a thought or opinion resulting from reflection

B. **Reflection**
  • Deliberation
  • Something provided by reflecting
  • A thought, idea or opinion formed or a remark made as a result of serious thought or consideration
  • Psychologically, turning one's mind upon experiences, percepts, ideas, etc. with a view to the discovery of new relations or the drawing of conclusions for the guidance of future action

Figure 7.1 Meanings of reflection

physical realm and the non-physical thinking mind. Reasoning is closely related to rationality; the term 'rational' is used to describe beliefs that are based upon appropriate reasons, whereas beliefs that do not conform to reason are termed 'irrational'. Evans and Over (1997) propose that the term 'rationality' is used in two different ways.

• Rationality 1 (personal rationality) is demonstrated in the successful achievement of basic life goals such as survival, communication with others and the ability to find one's way in the world.
• Rationality 2 (impersonal rationality) requires the ability to think hypothetically, i.e. to construct mental models to represent the world, and is typically demonstrated in decision-making and problem-solving.

Other constructs with similarities to reflection

Figure 7.2 gives a selection of constructs that share similarities with reflection.

• **Consciousness** refers to our awareness of internal and external phenomena including thoughts, emotions, sensations and moods. The term 'stream of consciousness' was coined by William James to describe an individual's perception of her/his own consciousness as continuously flowing and constantly changing awareness.
• **Cognition** refers to the mental processing or use of knowledge.
• **Thinking** has a number of diverse forms, such as reasoning, considering, deliberating and reflecting, and is closely related to language.
• **Metacognition** is 'thinking about thinking', i.e. it involves knowledge about one's own internal mental processes.
• **Introspection** involves 'looking into one's own mind'. An individual may ascertain both current and past mental states through introspection; the latter is termed 'retrospection' or 'recollection'.

Figure 7.2 Constructs similar to reflection

Critical thinking

Although critical thinking is another construct that is similar to reflection, it merits a separate discussion owing to the importance placed upon it in programmes for continuing professional development in nursing. Course documentation invariably contains some reference to the development of practitioner's skills of critical enquiry, analysis, critical awareness, critical thinking and evaluative skills. Definitions of critical thinking are not clear cut; for example, McBurney (1996) states 'I believe that critical thinking is primarily an attitude of asking why – why is that so? why did that happen? why should I believe that claim?' My own view is that critical thinking is best considered as a core concept consisting of a number of abilities (Quinn, 1995), as shown in Figure 7.3.

---

1. Ability to define a problem
2. Ability to select relevant information for problem-solving
3. Ability to draw inferences from observed or supposed facts
4. Ability to recognize assumptions
5. Ability to formulate relevant hypotheses
6. Ability to make deductions, i.e. draw conclusions from premises
7. Ability to make interpretations from data, i.e. judging whether or not a conclusion follows beyond a reasonable doubt from the facts given
8. Ability to evaluate arguments, i.e. to distinguish between strong arguments and weak arguments

---

Figure 7.3 Critical thinking abilities

There is some variation in the literature with regard to these components; Brookfield (1987), for example, identifies the following components.

- **Identifying and challenging assumptions**: Critical thinkers ask awkward questions in order to identify and challenge the assumptions which underlie issues and problems.
- **Challenging the importance of context**: Critical thinkers are aware that beliefs, actions, and established practice reflect the context in which they are set, both cultural and professional.
- **Imagining and exploring alternatives**: Critical thinkers have the ability to imagine and explore alternatives to established ways of thinking or behaving, because they are aware of the assumptions and the context of issues or problems.
- **Reflective scepticism**: Reflective thinkers take a sceptical view of established dogma and practices, carefully scrutinizing them and questioning their current validity.

Bloom's taxonomy: the cognitive domain

Since reflection is an intellectual or cognitive process, it may be helpful to refer to a long-established classification of levels of cognitive functioning: Bloom's taxonomy.

In his taxonomy of educational objectives Bloom (1956) identifies three domains of learning. The cognitive domain is concerned with knowledge and intellectual abilities, and provides an interesting classification of the various levels of intellectual functioning. There are six levels of objective and they are arranged in a hierarchy from level 1 at the bottom to level 6 at the top.

In a hierarchy, each level subsumes the ones below it; for example, in order for an individual to be able to engage in analysis, s/he must have the necessary intellectual prerequisites of knowledge, comprehension and application.

- **Level 1. Knowledge**: At this, the most basic level, all that is required is the bringing to mind of such things as specific facts or terminology.
- **Level 2. Comprehension**: This refers to understanding, which is usually demonstrated by the learner making limited use of the information, e.g. paraphrasing a communication while maintaining the intent of the original.
- **Level 3. Application**: The learner is required to apply rules, principles, concepts, etc. to real situations. These should be sufficiently unfamiliar to avoid the mere recall of previous behaviours.
- **Level 4. Analysis**: This involves the ability to break down information into its component parts, which may be elements of information, relationships between elements or organization and structure of information. Its purpose is to separate the important aspects of information from the less important, thus clarifying the meaning.
- **Level 5. Synthesis**: At this level the learner is required to combine various parts into a new kind of whole. Creativity is present because the learner produces something unique, such as a plan or design.
- **Level 6. Evaluation**: This implies the ability to make judgements regarding the value of material and involves the use of criteria.

The taxonomy offers a way of conceptualizing the different levels of intellectual functioning, and emphasizes the hierarchical way in which it is organized. The intellectual effort required for the recall of factual information is situated at the bottom of the intellectual hierarchy, while that required for evaluation or judgement is at the top. However, this does not imply that the lower levels are less important, simply that they are necessary prerequisites for higher-level intellectual functioning.

Where, then, does all this leave us in terms of a definition of reflection? From the foregoing discussion, I would suggest that the term is used in two ways:

- in a general sense, as synonymous with thinking and deliberating;
- in a specific sense, as the recollection of past experiences and mental states by retrospection. Indeed, the word reflection is derived from the Latin *reflectere* meaning 'to bend back'.

It is the latter use that is predominant within the literature of the nursing profession.

ARE MODELS OF REFLECTION HELPFUL FOR CLARIFYING WHAT REFLECTION IS?

Some models of reflection have established themselves as front-runners in nursing, particularly those of Kolb (1984), Schon (1983, 1987), Boud, Keogh and Walker (1985; Boud, Cohen and Walker, 1993) and Johns (1992). Models of reflection, while differing in their levels of explanation, envisage reflection as essentially a retrospective phenomenon consisting of three fundamental processes:

- **retrospection**: i.e. thinking back about a situation or experience;
- **self-evaluation**, i.e. critically analysing and evaluating the actions and feelings associated with the experience, using theoretical perspectives;
- **reorientation**, i.e. using the results of self-evaluation to influence future approaches to similar situations or experiences.

Kolb's experiential learning cycle

For David Kolb (1984) learning is a core process of human development that is clearly distinguishable from a simple readjustment to change. His experiential learning model (experiential learning cycle) is based upon the premise that development results from learning gained through experience. According to Kolb there are four generic adaptive abilities that are required for effective learning.

- **Concrete experience (CE):** The learner must immerse him/herself fully and openly in new experiences.
- **Reflective observation (RO):** The learner must observe and reflect on concrete experiences from a variety of perspectives.
- **Abstract conceptualization (AC):** The learner must create concepts that integrate his/her observations into logical theories.
- **Active experimentation:** The learner must apply these theories in decision-making and problem-solving.

These four generic adaptive abilities consist of two pairs of opposites, which together form two primary dimensions of learning:

Concrete experience —— Abstract conceptualization
Active experimentation —— Reflective observation

Figure 7.4 shows the reflective cycle. The cycle commences with a concrete experience, either professional or personal, that is perceived by the individual as interesting or problematic. Firstly, observations and information are gathered about the experience, and then the individual reflects upon it over and over again. By analysing this reflection, insights begin to emerge as a kind of 'theory' about the experience. Implications can then be drawn from this conceptualization and used to modify existing practice or to generate new approaches to practice. The

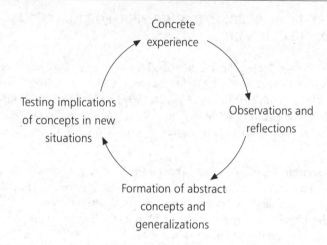

Figure 7.4 Kolb's experiential learning model

following example from professional nursing practice shows how the Kolb cycle
can be used as a vehicle for learning from experience.

KOLB'S CYCLE: EXAMPLE FROM PROFESSIONAL PRACTICE

Janice was a student nurse studying on the common foundation programme, and
was undertaking observations on a female surgical ward. It was lunchtime and she
saw a nurse deliver a meal to a patient; the meal was left untouched, so Janice
enquired of the patient why this was so. The patient told Janice that her arthritis
made it difficult to cut up her food, and she was hoping someone would come back
to do it for her. Janice duly obliged, and later on that day she pondered on why the
nurse who delivered the meal had not simply cut it up at the time. She went back
to the patient's bed and spent some time looking at the care plan; although it had
been meticulously maintained and updated, Janice realized that there was incon-
sistency between the intentions expressed in the care plan and the actual implementation of care. As she thought more and more about it, she recalled her
psychology lectures on human information processing and began to formulate a
sort of 'theory' about what had happened. Nurses practise in a busy and stressful
environment, bombarded with lots of information; coping strategies may therefore
develop that reduce information overload by focusing on routine procedural
aspects of care such as writing and updating care plans, to the detriment of observation of actual care being delivered. Hence, the failure of the nurse to cut up the
patient's meal was not an intentional act; rather, it was a failure to associate the
individual needs of the patient with the delivery of the meal. Janice realized that
she was also vulnerable to this problem, and resolved to maintain her focus on
patients and clients.

Kolb's model does not have a great deal of empirical support, however, and it is unlikely that all learning situations will require an integrated approach using the four generic adaptive abilities.

Boud, Keogh and Walker's model of reflection

The Boud, Keogh and Walker (1985) model is a three-stage model to assist learners to reflect upon experiences.

- **Stage 1. Returning to the experience**: In this stage the learner mentally 'replays' the experience, describing what happened in a descriptive, non-judgemental way.
- **Stage 2. Attending to feelings**: This stage is about getting in touch with the learner's own feelings about the experience, utilizing any positive feelings about the experience and removing any feelings that may obstruct the reflection.
- **Stage 3. Re-evaluating the experience**: This stage is broken down into four substages, each of which is designed to enhance outcomes of reflection. In re-evaluating the experience, it is important that any new information arising from experience and reflection makes an **association** with the learner's existing knowledge and attitudes. These associations are then put together by **integration** into new ideas or attitudes, which are then tested by **validation** to determine whether there are any inconsistencies or contradictions. The fourth substage, **appropriation**, occurs when the new knowledge and attitudes become an intrinsic part of the learner's identity, and this will depend upon the significance placed upon any given experience and associated reflections.

BOUD, KEOGH AND WALKER'S MODEL: EXAMPLE FROM PROFESSIONAL PRACTICE

Tara, a health visitor, was visiting a new mother in a block of flats. She had been asked by the university to take along a student nurse who was undertaking her community experience, and they parked the car outside. Tara knocked at the door of the flat and the mother opened the door. She was pleased to see Tara, whom she knew quite well, and after greeting the two visitors she asked: 'Are you going to weigh little Jamie today?' Tara explained that she had not intended to, so had left the scales in the car. Seeing the look of disappointment on the mother's face, she changed her mind and asked the student nurse if she would pop down to the car and fetch the scales. To her dismay the student replied 'No!' Somewhat disconcerted by this, Tara quickly said to the student, 'You stay here, and I'll fetch the scales'. After the visit had concluded, Tara and the student had a debriefing session in the car; Tara asked the student to explain her refusal and was told, 'It's not my job to carry weighing scales about'. On returning to base, Tara reported the student to tutorial staff at the university, and a disciplinary meeting was held involving Tara, the student, Tara's manager and the student's tutor. The student maintained that her reason for the refusal was that she was afraid she would not be able to turn off the car alarm; no further disciplinary action was taken.

Tara chose to reflect upon this experience using the Boud, Keogh and Walker model, and wrote the above description in her reflective diary. She found it difficult to attend to the feelings that were aroused by the incident; she felt that the student had behaved in a very unprofessional manner, particularly in front of a client, and she also resented being placed in such an embarrassing position herself. She couldn't help feeling that the only reason the disciplinary issue had not been pursued was because the student was a member of an ethnic minority, and that the university had wanted to avoid becoming embroiled in accusations of racism. The only positive feelings associated with the incident related to the fact that the mother had either missed or ignored the student's refusal and did not appear to have been affected by it. In trying to re-evaluate the experience, Tara tried to think of other past experiences that might shed light on the student's behaviour. She recalled that the student had changed her initial reason for refusing to collect the scales, subsequently citing fear of the car alarm as the motivating factor; perhaps there were cultural factors that could account for the student's reluctance to disclose the real reason for her refusal, such as the importance of not losing face in public. Tara did not have the opportunity to see the student again, but resolved to make sure that all students accompanying her on visits to clients' homes were fully briefed beforehand. However, she could still not see how the situation could have been anticipated in this case.

The Boud, Keogh and Walker model demonstrates a relatively rational approach to the process of reflecting upon experience, and as such as been adopted widely in nursing as a tool for teaching practitioners how to reflect. It is worth noting, however, that in a more recent paper (Boud, Cohen and Walker, 1993) the authors emphasize that systematic reflection is not the only way in which individuals learn from experiences:

> What we can say is that learning from experience is far more indirect than we often pretend it to be. It can be prompted by systematic reflection, but it can also be powerfully prompted by discrepancies or dilemmas which we are 'forced' to confront.

They go on to conclude:

> Much as we may enjoy the intellectual chase, we cannot neglect our full experience in the process. To do so is to fool ourselves into treating learning from experience as a simple, rational process.

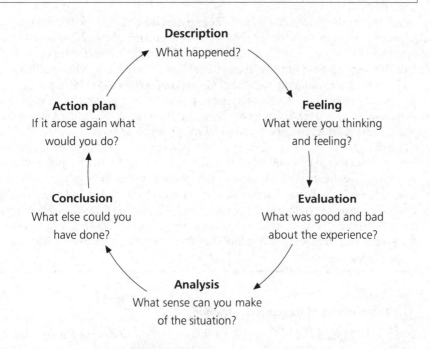

Figure 7.5 The Gibbs reflective cycle

The Gibbs reflective cycle

Figure 7.5 illustrates Gibbs's (1988) reflective cycle. It is interesting to note that, although at first sight it looks similar to the Kolb cycle, it is actually much closer to the Boud, Keogh and Walker model. Gibbs uses the term 'description' rather than 'returning to the experience'; the emphasis on dealing with good and bad feelings is similar in both cycles; Gibbs's term 'analysis' is less specific than 're-evaluating the experience' in the Boud *et al.* model, but in his reflective cycle Gibbs makes more overt the action planning component of reflection.

THE GIBBS REFLECTIVE CYCLE: EXAMPLE FROM PROFESSIONAL PRACTICE

Anne was a clinical nurse manager on a paediatric unit. A baby was admitted for assessment of feeding problems, but the medical and nursing staff could not find anything wrong with the baby's feeding. During discussion at the staff meeting, the nurses expressed the opinion that the mother had not been given adequate support by community staff and had therefore got herself into a 'muddle'; this had led to her perception that the baby was not feeding properly. Anne decided to ask the mother if she could look at her parent-held record, and noted that 12 entries had been made by the health visitor over a period of 2 months, which indicated a high level of support. Later in the week, Anne was writing up her reflective diary using the Gibbs reflective cycle as a framework. She recalled her feelings on discovering the high level of support given to the mother, noting that she felt annoyed and disappointed in her nursing staff for jumping to incorrect conclusions. However, there were also some good things about the experience, particularly the fact that she had looked for evidence of support from an objective source rather than relying on speculation. Anne then tried to put the situation into perspective; she concluded that the nurses had adopted a judgemental approach based entirely on their own perspective, rather than gathering all the available evidence before coming to a conclusion about the level of support. She analysed her own response to the situation and was pleased that she had been able to demonstrate the importance of evidence-based decision making, and this reinforced her view that she would adopt the same approach in the event of the experience happening again.

The Johns model of structured reflection

Johns (1992) uses the concept of guided reflection to describe a structured, supported approach that helps practitioners learn from their reflections upon experiences. The approach involves the use of the model of structured reflection, one-to-one or group supervision and the keeping of a structured reflective diary. The model of structured reflection involves a series of questions that help structure the practitioner's reflections. There is one core question and five cue questions, as shown in Figure 7.6.

Johns's model is more detailed than any of the models outlined above, and there are both advantages and disadvantages to this. The nursing literature indicates that nurses need to be taught how to reflect, and the detailed questions that practitioners are required to ask of themselves in the Johns model certainly provide a comprehensive checklist for reflection. The disadvantage of such a detailed structure is that it imposes a framework that is external to the practitioner, leaving little scope for inclusion of his/her own approach. It is also open to criticism on the grounds of complexity, although other models can be criticized on precisely the opposite grounds, i.e. they may appear simplistic and self-evident.

Stockhausen's clinical learning spiral

Stockhausen's (1994) clinical learning spiral has similarities to the Boud, Keogh and Walker model outlined earlier in the section. The focus of the spiral is undergraduate student nurses and it is designed to encourage the development of reflective practice in both students and their teachers. However, it is possible to speculate that the spiral might also act as a basis for continuing professional development.

Core question: What information do I need access to in order to learn through this experience?

Cue questions

1.0 *Description of experience*
    1.1 *Phenomenon* – describe the 'here and now' experience
    1.2 *Causal* – What essential factors contributed to this experience?
    1.3 *Context* – What are the significant background actors to this experience?
    1.4 *Clarifying* – What are the key processes (for reflection) in this experience?

2.0 *Reflection*
    2.1 What was I trying to achieve?
    2.2 Why did I intervene as I did?
    2.3 What were the consequences of my actions for:
      – Myself?
      – The patient/family?
      – The people I work with?
    2.4 How did I feel about this experience when it was happening?
    2.5 How did the patient feel about it?
    2.6 How do I know how the patient felt about it?

3.0 *Influencing factors*
    3.1 What internal factors influenced my decision making?
    3.2 What external factors influenced my decision making?
    3.3 What sources of knowledge did/should have influenced my decision making?

4.0 *Could I have dealt better with the situation?*
    4.1 What other choices did I have?
    4.2 What would be the consequences of those choices?

5.0 *Learning*
    5.1 How do I **now** feel about this experience?
    5.2 How have I made sense of this experience in the light of past experiences and future practice?
    5.3 How has this experience changed my ways of knowing:
      – empirics?
      – aesthetics?
      – ethics?
      – personal?

Figure 7.6 The Johns model of structured reflection

The notion of a spiral rather than a cyclical process allows for progressively deeper levels to be attained, and the number of spirals that may occur is limitless. Each consists of four phases, as shown in Figure 7.7.

The preparative phase, as the name suggests, is concerned with preparation for clinical experience and involves campus-based learning in classroom and nursing skills laboratory, and also a briefing session prior to the beginning of a placement experience. This offers the opportunity for students to discuss their forthcoming experience and to share any anxieties they may have. The constructive phase refers

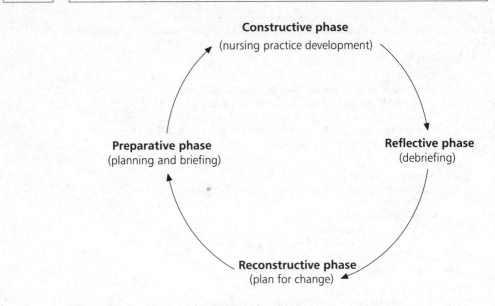

Figure 7.7 Stockhausen's clinical learning spiral

to all the facets of the student's clinical placement experience, including the development of nursing skills and interventions and the evaluation of care. This is followed by the reflective phase, in which the student undergoes debriefing and constructive feedback, in both one-to-one and group settings. This phase is very much based on the Boud, Keogh and Walker model, and provides the students with the opportunity to share experiences and feelings with teachers and peers. The final stage, reconstruction, is concerned with planning for change on the basis of the reflections of the previous stage and incorporates goal-setting prior to taking action to address the changes. The four phases of the spiral can be applied to learning at both preregistration and postregistration levels; the differences for the latter will be most evident in the content of the constructive phase and in the depth of experience brought to bear in the reflective practice phase.

From the foregoing review of a range of models of reflection from both the teaching and the nursing professions, it is clear that reflection is interpreted predominantly as retrospection or reflection after an experience. Although these models of reflection differ in their approach, there is general agreement about the conscious and goal-directed nature of reflection, and the inter-relationship between its intellectual and emotional aspects.

WHAT IS MEANT BY 'REFLECTIVE PRACTICE' AND WHY IS IT IMPORTANT?

Reflective practice as the dominant model in nursing

The concept of reflective practice has been adopted by the nursing profession as the dominant model for professional practice. The UKCC postregistration education and practice requirements endorse the importance of reflection in the requirement that every practitioner maintains a personal professional profile. The profile 'is based on a regular process of reflection and recording what you learn from everyday experiences, as well as planned learning activity' (UKCC, 1997). Reflection is also a key component of clinical supervision; in its position paper on clinical supervision, the UKCC makes six key statements, the first of which states: 'Clinical supervision supports practice, enabling practitioners to **maintain and promote standards of care**'. The rationale for this statement is given as 'By encouraging reflection on practice issues, the practitioner's skills, knowledge and professional values will be enhanced and career development and lifelong learning will be promoted' (UKCC, 1996). Although reflection is not specifically mentioned in the UKCC Code of Conduct (UKCC, 1992), Palmer (1994) draws the inference that:

> it could be suggested that it will be the responsibility of each practising nurse, midwife and health visitor to introduce reflection into their professional practice if reflection is considered a necessary requisite for the evaluation and development of professional practice.

Approaches to reflective practice

Pinning down the concept of reflective practice is not straightforward; definitions in the literature range from the relatively simple, e.g. 'The concept of reflective practice is mainly associated with the idea of reflection on experience' (Johns, 1996a), to the more complex, e.g.:

> reflective practice then is more than just thoughtful practice, it is the process of turning thoughtful practice into a potential learning situation and, significantly enough, it is the utilization of good theory in practice in what must always be a situation of probability – but the professional reflective practitioner is always trying to ensure that the outcome of any action is close to what is anticipated by the theory and the previous experience combined. (Jarvis, 1992)

Schon: The Reflective Practitioner

Perhaps the single most influential interpretation of reflective practice is that of Donald Schon, whose approach has influenced thinking about professional practice in a number of professions, not least those of teaching and nursing.

The publication of Donald Schon's book *The Reflective Practitioner: How Professionals Think in Action* (Schon, 1983) has had a considerable impact on both the teaching and the nursing professions, providing as it does an alternative rationale for professional practice.

Schon's focus is the relationship between academic knowledge as defined in universities and the competence involved in professional practice. He argues that professional practice is based upon a technical rationality model that makes erroneous assumptions about the nature of practice, and in so doing reduces its importance in relation to theory. Technical rationality views professional practice as the application of general, standardized, theoretical principles to the solving of practice problems; in other words, professional practice is problem-solving. This top-down view puts general theoretical principles at the top of the hierarchy of professional knowledge and practical problem-solving at the bottom, leading to what Schon termed the pre-eminence of theory and the denigration of practice.

Problem-setting
Within the technical rationality model, professional practice is viewed as a process of instrumental problem-solving, with the assumption that problems are self-evident. Schon, however, argues that in reality practitioners are not presented with problems *per se*, but with problem situations. These must be converted into actual problems by a process of problem-setting, i.e. selecting the elements of the situation, deciding the ends and means and framing the context. Technical rationality also fails to take account of the fact that problems encountered in professional practice are rarely standard or predictable.

Knowing-in-action
Schon uses this term to describe the intuitive or tacit 'knowing' that is embedded in professional actions. Intuition is a mental process commonly termed 'the sixth sense', and refers to a process by which an individual comes to a conclusion about something in the absence of sensory inputs and without consciously thinking about it. For example, skilled practitioners constantly make intuitive judgements about situations without being able to specify exactly the criteria they base those judgements on; this is often termed 'thinking on your feet'. Schon maintains that, although this intuitive 'knowing' is implicit within our actions, it is possible for practitioners to access this by reflecting on what they are doing while they are doing it.

Reflection-in-action
Reflection-in-action occurs when the practitioner is confronted by a novel puzzle or problem situation which s/he attempts to resolve. This resolution occurs when

the problem is **re-framed**, i.e. seen differently during the actions. The process of reflecting upon the intuitive 'knowing' that is implicit in a practitioner's actions, while at the same time carrying out those actions, together constitutes reflection-in-action.

It is important to emphasize that the reflection is inherent in the action itself, and not in any thinking going on at the same time. Reflection-in-action is non-rational and non-linear, and is embedded in the action. Richardson (1990) succinctly captures this phenomenon: 'Schon found intelligence in the act itself rather than in attempting to make the act seem intelligent'. Schon suggests that reflection-in-action is triggered more commonly by surprising results, whereas anticipated results are less likely to be thought about. Reflection-in-action occurs within what Schon terms the action-present, i.e. the timescale in which any action by the practitioner can still influence a situation.

Reflection-on-action
This is the type of reflection that is referred to in the models of reflection discussed in the previous section of this chapter and involves retrospection on past experiences, the aim of which is to generate knowledge for future practice. Reflection-on-action contrasts markedly with reflection-in-action, the latter occurring while the practitioner is engaged in actions rather than thinking about it later.

Knowledge-in-action
This is practical professional knowledge, and develops by the process of reflection-in-action. It does not rely on a series of conscious steps in a decision-making process; instead it is inherent in the action itself. It is not possible to ascertain this knowledge-in-action by talking to a practitioner, as it is not a conscious process, but expert knowledge can be elicited by observing the practitioner reflecting-in-action.

Characteristics of reflective practitioners
This notion of the reflective practitioner, according to Schon, contrasts markedly with the prevailing model of professional practice, the technical rationality model.

According to Schon, the reflective practitioner is characterized by a range of personal qualities and abilities, such as the ability to engage in self-assessment; to criticize the existing state of affairs; to promote change and to adapt to change; to practise as an autonomous professional. He also distinguishes between the effective and the ineffective practitioner: the former is able to recognize and explore confusing or unique events that occur during practice, whereas the latter is 'burned-out', i.e. confined to repetitive and routine practice, neglecting opportunities to think about what s/he is doing

Although Schon's ideas on reflective practice have been widely accepted within the nursing profession, his approach has been criticized for a lack of empirical support. Munby and Russell (1989) point out that there is 'virtually no elaboration of the psychological realities of reflection-in-action', e.g. What makes it begin? What happens when it begins? How do we know when it is occurring?

Benner: From Novice to Expert

It is interesting to compare Benner's approach to the development of expert practice with the views of Schon on reflective practice. In her book *From Novice to Expert*, Benner (1984) described the characteristics of performance at five different levels of nursing skill: novice, advanced beginner, competent, proficient and expert. (Benner uses the term skill in its widest sense to mean all aspects of nursing practice, and not simply psychomotor skill performance.) During his/her passage through these stages, the student relies less upon abstract rules to govern his/her practice and more on his/her past experience. Nursing situations begin to be seen as a unified whole within which only certain aspects are relevant, and the nurse becomes personally involved in situations rather than a detached observer. Hence, there are some similarities to Schon's approach, in particular the emphasis on the role of experience and the importance of intuition.

Stage 1: Novice

This level is characterized by rule-governed behaviour, as the novice has no experience of the situation upon which to draw, and this applies to both students in training and to experienced nurses who move into an unfamiliar clinical area. Adherence to principles and rules, however, does not help the nurse to decide what is relevant in a nursing situation, and may thus lead to unsuccessful performance.

Stage 2: Advanced beginner

Unlike principles and rules, aspects are overall characteristics of a situation that can only be identified by experience of that situation. For example, the skills of interviewing a patient are developed by experience of interviewing previous patients, and the advanced beginner is one who has had sufficient prior experience of a situation to deliver marginally acceptable performance. Advanced beginners need adequate support from supervisors, mentors and colleagues in the practice setting.

Stage 3: Competent

This stage is characterized by conscious, deliberate planning based upon analysis and careful deliberation of situations. The competent nurse is able to identify priorities and manage his/her work, and Benner suggests that s/he can benefit at this stage from learning activities that centre on decision-making, planning and coordinating patient care.

Stage 4: Proficient

Unlike the competent nurse, the proficient nurse has the ability to home in directly on the most relevant aspects of a problem, because s/he is able to perceive situations holistically. According to Benner, proficient performance is based upon the use of maxims, and is normally found in nurses who have worked within a specific area of nursing for several years. Inductive teaching strategies, such as case studies, are most useful for nurses at this stage.

Stage 5: Expert

This stage is characterized by a deep understanding and intuitive grasp of the total situation; the expert nurse develops a feel for situations and a vision of the possibilities in a given situation. The expert is able to bring his/her intuition to bear on practice, rather than doing everything 'by the book'. Benner suggests that critical incident technique is a useful way of attempting to evaluate expert practice, but also that not all nurses are capable of becoming experts.

Perspectives on reflective practice from the literature of teacher education

The following perspectives are taken from the literature of teacher education, but are useful in providing the views of another profession on the nature of reflective practice. Hill (1996) contrasts the attributes of reflective and non-reflective practitioners:

> [N]on-reflective teachers rely on routine behaviour and are guided more by impulse, tradition and authority than by reflection. They simplify their professional lives, uncritically accepting everyday reality in schools. In contrast, reflective teachers actively, persistently and carefully consider and reconsider beliefs and practices.

Grimmett et al.: Three Perspectives on Reflective Practice

Grimmett *et al.* (1990), also writing about reflective practice in the context of teacher education, offer three perspectives.

1. **Reflection as instrumental mediation of action**: In this 'top-down' perspective, the practitioner reflects upon relevant theory and research and then applies it to professional practice. Hence, the practitioner's knowledge **directs** his/her practice.
2. **Reflection as deliberating among competing views (of teaching)**: In choosing between competing views of practice, the practitioner utilizes relevant theory and research. However, in this perspective, reflection involves deliberating about these in the light of the context of practice and the opinions of colleagues before reaching a decision. Hence, the practitioner's knowledge **informs** his/her practice.
3. **Reflection as reconstructing experience**: In this perspective, puzzlement and subsequent reflection about situations in professional practice lead to new knowledge in the form of insights and understandings about the situation.

In this case, the practitioner's knowledge **transforms** his/her practice.

These three perspectives can be seen to relate closely to Schon's ideas about professional practice, moving from a technical rationality approach in perspective 1 to that of reflective practice in perspective 3.

Wellington and Austin: Five Orientations to Reflective Practice

According to Wellington and Austin, reflective practitioners think and write about things they perceive as practical. From their analysis of a large number of reflective journal entries written by practising teachers, they suggest five orientations to reflective practice, as outlined in Figure 7.8. For each orientation, the practitioner's typical characteristics and reflective writing are proposed.

While Wellington and Austin's approach does not appear at first glance to have any relevance for CPD in nursing, on closer inspection a number of the characteristics could well apply to some practitioners in nursing. The link between individual characteristics and reflective writing in each orientation is particularly interesting.

WHAT OTHER STRATEGIES CAN BE USED TO FACILITATE REFLECTION?

Reflective writing

Reflective writing is the term given to a range of written reflections including profiling, portfolios, reflective journals, reflective diaries, personal letters and narratives. Reflective writing, in this sense, refers to the retrospective analysis of past experiences, and comprises an important learning strategy in nurse education at both preregistration and postregistration levels. One of the values of reflective writing is that the record is permanently available for further reflection on future occasions. Reflective writing, in the form of a personal professional portfolio, is one of the UKCC's PREPP requirements for continuing registration (UKCC, 1997). Personal professional portfolios are discussed in detail in Chapter 9.

Critical incident analysis

Critical incident technique (Flanagan, 1954) provides a useful strategy for helping practitioners to reflect. Benner, in her study of the acquisition of nursing skill cited earlier in this chapter, identified critical incidents in nursing as comprising any of the following:

- those in which the nurse's intervention really made a difference in patient outcome;
- those that went unusually well;

Characteristics of reflective practitioners and their reflective writing:

1. **Immediate orientation**
   - Emphasis is on pleasant survival
   - Ready acceptance of the status quo
   - Tend to focus on the immediate task in hand
   - Teaching is often eclectic but shallow
   - Likely to use any methodology that seems promising in a particular situation

   Reflective writing is simple reporting, and essentially non-reflective

2. **Technical orientation**
   - Focuses primarily on classroom unit
   - Typically emphasizes behaviourist techniques
   - Functions in a diagnostic/prescriptive mode

   Reflective writing emphasizes the correct execution of preconceived teaching methods

3. **Deliberative orientation**
   - Emphasis on discovery, assignment and assessment of personal meaning
   - May feel uncomfortable at times working in authorized organizational structures
   - May negotiate with authorities for changes in academic content
   - Concern extends beyond the classroom, helping individuals to discover personal relevance within the institutional structure

   Reflective writing often brings tacit assumption into awareness

4. **Dialectic orientation**
   - Reject the limitations of authorized organizational structures and are uncomfortable working within them
   - Question educational aims, content and means
   - Tend to focus on political and social issues
   - Teaching involves continual questioning, revision and internal validation
   - Stresses empowerment and personal responsibility
   - Is contextually sensitive and responsive

   Reflective writing grapples with ways to create justice and equity in education and society

5. **Transpersonal orientation**
   - Centre on universal personal liberation
   - Resist the imposed restraints of authorized organizational structures
   - Focus on self-development
   - Teaching is typically individualized and holistic

   Reflective writing is introspective and often highly personal

Figure 7.8 Orientations to reflective practice (Wellington and Austin, 1996)

- those in which there was a breakdown;
- those that were ordinary and typical;
- those that captured the essence of nursing;
- those that were particularly demanding.

Benner's study provides a useful framework for reflecting upon and analysing critical incidents, leading to new insights into practice; descriptions of critical incidents should cover the following:

- the context of the incident;
- a detailed description of it;
- why the incident was critical to the practitioner;
- what the practitioner's concerns were at the time;
- what s/he was thinking about during the incident;
- what s/he felt about it afterwards;
- what s/he found most demanding about it.

Wood (1998) offers a four-stage model for analysing critical incidents:

- **Stage 1**: description of what took place during the incident;
- **Stage 2**: analysis of communication skills used and clarification of the under-pinning moral values;
- **Stage 3**: exploration of potentially effective alternative strategies to those skills actually employed, including moral justification for proposed alternatives;
- **Stage 4**: identification of implications for practice.

Critical incident technique is not without its problems; Rich and Parker (1995) explore the morality of using critical incident technique as a teaching and learning tool. They point out that if students' critical incidents contain reference to dangerous behaviour or unprofessional conduct, the tutor or lecturer may be deemed to be in breach of the UKCC code of conduct if s/he does not report the behaviour to the appropriate authorities.

Clinical supervision

Clinical supervision is a concept of growing importance within nursing. Faugier and Butterworth (1994) define it as 'an exchange between practising profession-als to enable the development of professional skills'. Reflection upon experience is a central component of clinical supervision, and the process of reflection is facil-itated by the presence of a supervisor. Clinical supervision is discussed in detail in Chapter 8.

ARE THERE ANY RESERVATIONS EXPRESSED ABOUT REFLECTIVE PRACTICE?

It seems self-evident that, by reflecting upon practice, practitioners may gain insights into how their practice can be improved. Indeed, it is probably impossi-ble to avoid reflecting on the past, particularly when the recollected situation or event has emotional overtones for the practitioner.

However, I would like to express some reservations I have about the way in which it is being promulgated in nursing. The impression gained from the literature is that the only effective nurses are those who actively and systematically reflect upon their practice, and that such reflection must be more than simply thinking about the situation or event. I have categorized my reservations under three headings: ethical, professional and pragmatic.

Ethical reservations

The theoretical basis for reflection, as interpreted by the nursing profession, is humanistic psychology as exemplified in the work of Carl Rogers (1951, 1969, 1983). It is therefore from the same stable as interpersonal skills training, encounter groups, and assertiveness training, all of which emphasize the paramouncy of the **self** and the importance of **feelings** over cognition, e.g. self-awareness, self-disclosure, self-actualization.

Criticism of this 1960s 'pop psychology' is beginning to emerge; Sigman (1995) suggests that during this period psychology diversified from the treating of problems to addressing issues of greater happiness. He argues that individuals' expectations turned away from contentment and self-acceptance towards personal growth and development. This constant striving for self-improvement may lead to feelings of self-disapproval and rejection of one's own personality, especially if the individual fails to achieve the self-improvement s/he is seeking.

The nursing literature suggests that reflection is more valuable if done in partnership with someone else, which leads me to believe that the approach is quasi-therapeutic: in other words, the principles have been transferred directly from client-centred psychotherapy and Rogersian counselling. The examples of reflective encounters given by Johns (1996b) seem to me to be very much in this therapeutic mould.

The use of this approach may trigger powerful emotional responses such as guilt and anxiety, and as such we have to consider whether or not practitioners should be given a choice about participating in such activity.

Student nurses certainly appear to have no choice, as reflection is now a significant component of their preregistration education. The following quotation from Fitzgerald (1994, p. 76) is illuminating in this respect: 'These are not particularly comfortable processes, which may lead students to personal distress and conflict'. Other writers, e.g. Rich and Parker (1995), identify the unease of some students with this approach.

Qualified practitioners too may have little choice, since reflection is seen as a crucial component of clinical supervision (Fisher, 1996) and of the PREPP portfolio (UKCC, 1997). The question of choice is important also, given that there is currently little evidence for the effectiveness of reflective practice in nursing; indeed, the nature of reflective practice makes it almost impossible to evaluate with any accuracy. It is somewhat ironic, given the importance that nurses attach to informed consent in relation to patients and clients, that this aspect may have been entirely overlooked in the case of nursing staff and students.

It is interesting to note that the teaching profession, in its adoption of reflective practice, has placed much less emphasis on the emotional aspects of reflection, preferring instead to focus on the cognitive. This may well be because of the different goals and professional socialization of the two professions.

Professional reservations

The concept of victim-blaming is well established in the field of health promotion and refers to approaches that focus on the individual as the prime cause of his/her own ill-health, as opposed to the social, economic and political environment in which s/he lives. Similarly, reflective practice seems to put the onus on to the individual practitioner for the maintenance and improvement of standards of nursing care, which may divert attention away from the responsibility of the organization to provide adequate staffing levels, effective staff development and adequate resources.

Another difficulty I find is that the literature of reflective practice seems to constantly devalue current nursing practice, thus undermining both the individual practitioner and the nurse manager. It is interesting to note that most of the literature on clinical supervision suggests that the clinical supervisor should not be the individual practitioner's line manager, yet it is the latter who carries ultimate responsibility for the quality of care in a given practice context. This seems to imply that managers are not to be trusted, yet most nursing managers are themselves practitioners.

Relationships between nurse academics in colleges of nursing and practitioners in the field have been characterized by 'mutual distrust, little respect for each others' experience, even less empathy for each other, and often overt antagonism between the parties' (Quinn, 1994). The constant devaluing of current practice may undermine practitioners' confidence and lower their morale, resulting in a fall in standards of care, i.e. the exact opposite effect to what is intended by reflective practice.

Current models of reflective practice may also devalue physical care by overemphasizing psychological aspects. It is interesting to note that the devaluing of professional practice does not seem to occur to anything like the same extent in the literature of the teaching profession, which may lead one to conclude that the nursing profession may be going overboard in its critical approach to practice.

One could also advance the argument that reflection, particularly that done in partnership with a colleague or supervisor, could lead to the practitioner becoming dependent upon that individual, a well-documented phenomenon in the literature of counselling.

Pragmatic reservations

While reflection seems to be an important strategy for analysing individuals' practice, I have reservations about the practical implementation as proposed in the nursing literature. It is my belief that nurses already have too many professional development demands placed upon them, all of which are additional to their role in caring for patients. For example, nurses are required to engage in the following activities:

• maintain a PREPP portfolio as evidence for reregistration;

- undergo clinical supervision;
- undergo individual performance review (IPR) or appraisal;
- undertake statutory training, e.g. moving and handling;
- keep up to date by reading journals.

Given that current nursing practice is demanding, stressful and constantly changing, it may well be unfair and unrealistic to expect practitioners to reflect systematically on their practice unless they are given the time to do it during their working day. To quote one practitioner: 'After a hard day at work, the last thing I want to do when I get home is to start reflecting about it'. In the case of student nurses, there is also the potential for complicity, i.e. if written reflection is made a compulsory and assessed component of their education programme, students may invent reflections that meet the criteria laid down by their teachers.

The inference could be drawn that, if you are not a reflective practitioner in the way the term is interpreted in the nursing literature, you are not a good practitioner. Does this mean that practice was never any good before reflection was invented? It needs to be remembered that reflection, according to the nursing literature, is *ex post facto* and as such cannot affect the outcome of the situation being reflected upon. In effect, it can be seen as 'shutting the stable door after the horse has bolted'.

Of course, such reflection may influence the practitioner's approach to future situations, but this is a much less direct effect. What is needed, I suggest, is a shift of emphasis towards reflection-in-action and even reflection-before-action. Perhaps nurse education needs to emphasize much more the fact that nurses need not always respond to situations by 'thinking on their feet'. This can often lead to 'knee-jerk' reactions rather than carefully thought out responses. It is probably true to say that many situations in nursing do not require an instant response, and nurses might well benefit from the concept of 'taking time out' before making decisions in practice.

I am inclined to conclude that reflection as described in the literature should be seen as a strategy for student learning rather than a system for use by qualified practitioners in their everyday work. On the other hand, reflective cycles, e.g. Kolb (1984), Gibbs (1988), seem helpful, but can be done mentally without having to write everything down. However, to expect qualified, busy practitioners to be doing it on a regular basis is unwarranted given the present lack of evidence about its effectiveness. It is simply unacceptable for nurses to be branded as ineffective because they do not undertake the systematic process of reflection espoused by the proponents of reflective practice. Jarvis (1992) fired an early warning shot when he wrote: 'It might even be claimed that the idea of reflective practice is a band-wagon, upon which many professionals have jumped because it provides a rationale for their practice'. Richardson (1990) also counsels against 'the danger of taking an abstract concept like reflection, and operationalizing it into behaviour that is generalizable, observable and teachable'. At the time of writing, another concept is beginning to dominate the world of health care – evidence-based practice. It remains to be seen what effect, if any, this will have on current notions of reflective practice.

REFERENCES

Benner, P. (1984) *From Novice to Expert: Excellence and Power in Clinical Nursing Practice,* Addison-Wesley, Menlo Park, CA.

Bloom, B. (1956) *Taxonomy of Educational Objectives: The Classification of Educational Goals, Handbook 1: Cognitive Domain,* McKay, New York.

Boud, D., Cohen, R. and Walker, D. (eds) (1993) *Using Experience for Learning,* Open University Press, Milton Keynes.

Boud, D., Keogh, R. and Walker, D. (1985) *Reflection: Turning Experience into Learning,* Kogan Page, London.

Brookfield, S. (1987) *Developing Critical Thinkers,* Open University Press, Milton Keynes.

Evans, J. and Over, D. (1997) Are people rational? Yes, no and sometimes. *Psychologist,* **10**(9), 403–406.

Faugier, J. and Butterworth, T. (1994) *Clinical Supervision: A Positional Paper,* School of Nursing, University of Manchester, Manchester.

Fisher, M. (1996) Using reflective practice in clinical supervision. *Professional Nurse,* **11**(7), 443–444.

Fitzgerald, M. (1994) Theories of reflection for learning, in *Reflective Practice in Nursing,* (eds A. Palmer, S. Burns and C. Bulman), Blackwell, Oxford.

Flanagan, J. (1954) The critical incident technique. *Psychological Bulletin,* **51**, 327–358.

Gibbs, G. (1988) *Learning by Doing: A Guide to Teaching and Learning Methods,* Further Education Unit, Oxford Polytechnic, Oxford.

Gregory, R. L. (ed.) (1987) *The Oxford Companion to the Mind,* Oxford University Press, Oxford.

Grimmett, P., Erickson, G., Mackinnon, A. and Reicken, T. (1990) Reflective practice in teacher education, in *Encouraging Reflective Practice in Education,* (eds T. Clift, W. Houston and M. Pugach), Teachers College Press, New York.

Hill, J. (1996) Loopy learning – reflections on reflective practice. *Reflect,* **2**(2), 21–26.

Jarvis, P. (1992) Reflective practice and nursing, *Nurse Education Today,* **12**(3), 174–181.

Johns, C. (1992) The Burford Nursing Development Unit holistic model of nursing practice. *Journal of Advanced Nursing,* **16**, 1090–1098.

Johns, C. (1996a) Using a reflective model of nursing and guided reflection, *Nursing Standard,* **11**(2), 34–38.

Johns, C. (1996b) The benefits of a reflective model of nursing. *Nursing Times,* **92**, 27.

Kolb, D. A. (1984) *Experiential Learning,* Prentice-Hall, London

McBurney, D. (1996) *How to Think Like a Psychologist: Critical Thinking in Psychology,* Prentice-Hall, Englewood Cliffs, NJ.

Munby, H. and Russell, T. (1989) Educating the reflective teacher: an essay review of two books by Donald Schon. *Journal of Curriculum Studies,* **21**(1), 71–80.

Palmer, A. (1994) Introduction, in *Reflective Practice in Nursing: The Growth of the Professional Practitioner,* (eds A. Palmer, S. Burns and C. Bulman), Blackwell, Oxford.

Quinn, F. M. (1994) The demise of curriculum, in *Healthcare Education: The Challenge of the Market,* (eds J. Humphreys and F. M. Quinn), Chapman & Hall, London.

Quinn, F. M. (1995) *The Principles and Practice of Nurse Education*, 3rd edn, Stanley Thornes, Cheltenham.

Rich, A. and Parker, D. (1995) Reflection and critical incident analysis: ethical and moral implications of their use within nursing and midwifery education. *Journal of Advanced Nursing*, **22**, 1050–1057.

Richardson, V. (1990) The evolution of reflective teaching and teacher education, in *Encouraging Reflective Practice in Education*, (eds T. Clift, W. Houston and M. Pugach), Teachers College Press, New York.

Rogers, C. (1969) *Freedom to Learn*, Charles E. Merrill, Columbus, OH.

Rogers, C. (1983) *Freedom to Learn for the 80s*, Charles E. Merrill, Columbus, OH.

Rogers, C. (1951) *Client Centred Therapy*, Houghton Mifflin, Boston, MA.

Schon, D. (1983) *The Reflective Practitioner: How Professionals Think in Action*, Basic Books, New York.

Schon, D. (1987) *Educating the Reflective Practitioner: Towards a New Design for Teaching and Learning in the Professions*, Jossey-Bass, San Francisco, CA.

Sigman, A. (1995) *New, Improved? Exposing the Misuse of Popular Psychology*, Simon & Schuster, London.

Stockhausen, L. (1994) The clinical learning spiral: a model to develop reflective practitioners. *Nurse Education Today*, **14**(5), 363–371.

UKCC (1992) *Code of Professional Conduct for the Nurse, Midwife and Health Visitor*, 3rd edn, United Kingdom Central Council for Nursing, Midwifery and Health Visiting, London.

UKCC (1996) *Position Statement on Clinical Supervision for Nursing and Health Visiting*, United Kingdom Central Council for Nursing, Midwifery and Health Visiting, London.

UKCC (1997) *PREP and You*, United Kingdom Central Council for Nursing, Midwifery and Health Visiting, London.

Wellington, B. and Austin, P. (1996) Orientations to reflective practice. *Educational Research*, **38**(3), 307–316.

Wood, S. (1998) Ethics and communication: developing reflective practice. *Nursing Standard*, **12**(18), 44–47.

8	**Clinical supervision**

Pat Grant and Francis M. Quinn

INTRODUCTION

The concept of clinical supervision is now firmly established within nursing and health visiting, being perceived by the profession as an important vehicle for the professional development of its practitioners. Although not yet a statutory requirement for nurses, clinical supervision has been endorsed by the United Kingdom Central Council for Nursing, Midwifery and Health Visiting as 'an important part of strategies to promote high standards of nursing and health visiting care into the next century' (UKCC, 1996a). The Code of Professional Conduct (UKCC, 1992) states that 'as a registered nurse, midwife or health visitor you are personally accountable for your practice', and this principle relates directly to the aims of clinical supervision. The UKCC position paper on clinical supervision (UKCC, 1996a) sets out six key statements that highlight the nature and process of clinical supervision, the need for every practitioner to have access to it, the importance of training for supervisors and the need for evaluation at local level. A UKCC report on professional conduct complaints (UKCC, 1996b) notes that:

> in some cases [of professional misconduct] it is apparent that there are no systems in place to identify practitioners who are having difficulties. A systematic process of support and supervision should be in place and may help to identify problems.

The perceived importance of clinical supervision is eloquently expounded by Swain (1995):

> [A]ny one of us looking back at the human pain and social distress of others to which we have been exposed, not to mention our own, must surely question

what makes us suppose we can practise effectively without such a regular, conscientious examination of our work, of what might improve it and what impedes it, and of our own feelings about it.

Definitions of clinical supervision are plentiful within the literature; Faugier and Butterworth (1994) define it as 'an exchange between practising professionals to enable the development of professional skills'. This definition takes as its focus the development of the professional. Another definition, in the Department of Health document *Vision of the Future* (1993), incorporated the professional development focus as well as a client focus and stated that clinical supervision was:

a formal process of professional support and learning which enables the individual practitioner to develop knowledge and competence, assume responsibility for their own practice and enhance consumer protection and safety of care in complex clinical situations.

This definition by the Department of Health underpins the aims of supervision, which Bishop (1994) said were to:

- support the delivery of optimum care;
- safeguard standards;
- develop professional expertise.

Proctor's (1991) interactive model of supervision proposes three interactive functions of clinical supervision: formative, restorative and normative. The formative or educational function of clinical supervision is concerned with developing the knowledge and skills of the practitioner. The restorative function is about supporting the practitioner, particularly in those aspects of high emotional stress encountered in nursing practice.
Davies (1993) suggests that:

supervision says: this time is for you, you are worth it. That in itself has to be one way of reducing emotional pain and staff burn-out; cheaper than sickness, absenteeism and quick staff turnover.

The third function, normative, relates to quality assurance aspects of practice to ensure professional standards of care.
Figure 8.1 identifies the key characteristics of clinical supervision culled from the literature.
Clinical supervision shares some similarities with mentorship and preceptorship, but the overall aim is different, as are the roles of individuals undertaking these. One definition of a mentor is that of the ENB (1993):

an appropriately qualified and experienced first level nurse/midwife/health visitor who, by example and facilitation, guides, assists and supports the student in learning new skills, adopting new behaviour and acquiring new attitudes.

Purpose
- Professional support and learning
- Development of knowledge and competence
- Responsibility for own practice
- Enhance consumer protection
- Help practitioner to examine and validate his/her practice and feelings
- Pastoral support
- Formative assessment
- Ensuring standard of clinical and managerial practice
- Maintain and support standards of care
- To help the client
- Improve quality of patient care
- Improve staff performance
- Reduce stress and burn-out

Process
- A formal process
- A practice-focused professional relationship
- Should be developed according to local circumstances
- Every practitioner should have access
- Preparation for supervisors is important and should be included in pre- and postregistration programmes
- Evaluation is needed and should be determined locally

Figure 8.1 Characteristics of clinical supervision

It has been suggested (Armitage and Burnard, 1991) that preceptorship is more concerned with the teaching, learning and role-modelling aspects of the relationship, whereas mentorship is primarily about a close, personal relationship with the student. Quinn (1995) defines a preceptor as:

> an experienced nurse, midwife or health visitor within a practice placement who acts as a role model and resource for a student who is attached to her for a specific time-span or experience.

The aims of clinical supervision may not be fully achieved if managers attempt to provide it for their own staff. The main reason for this is conflict of roles. A manager's job involves staff appraisal and most practitioners want to be appraised positively, so it is unlikely that they will share the most vulnerable parts of their work with someone who is going to appraise them. Indeed, the work that is shared is likely to be the good bits, i.e. those parts that will impress the manager. What managers have to offer to their staff is managerial supervision, i.e. a type of supervision that allows managers to ensure that organizational policies are being put into practice, check on staff workload and facilitate mutual feedback. Managerial supervision is important but it should not be confused with clinical supervision. This perspective is underlined by the UKCC:

> [C]linical supervision is not a managerial control system. It is not, therefore, the exercise of overt managerial responsibility or managerial supervision;

not a system of formal individual performance review, or hierarchical in nature. (UKCC, 1996a)

However, Fisher (1996) describes a system of clinical supervision by line managers in a hospice setting which 'has been welcomed as appropriate', and McGibbon (1996) describes a similar system within the Ear, Nose and Throat specialism in which ward managers acted as clinical supervisors and 'encountered no significant problems'.

Clinical supervision has many benefits, some of which are improved patient care, dissemination of good practice, reduced staff turnover and job satisfaction (Bishop, 1994). Bishop also mentioned 'cost-effective use of training/education budget' as another benefit, but this needs to be interpreted with caution because, while it is true that clinical supervision does provide training/education, it is not a replacement for organized education/training. One would not want an organization to think that by investing in clinical supervision they have fulfilled their responsibility for training/education. Clinical supervision is only one factor in aiding professional development and providing quality care.

PREPARING FOR CLINICAL SUPERVISION

The literature of clinical supervision makes a clear distinction between the role and skills required of a supervisor and those of a supervisee, but it is important to remember that supervisors will also be supervisees, and *vice versa*. Hence, in many clinical supervision relationships, the participants will be experienced in both roles, which should normally facilitate the effectiveness of the process.

The supervisor

Like nursing, supervision occurs within a relationship, so all supervisors must have skills in building relationships. According to Atherton (1986), 'the quality of the supervisor's listening is the best guide to the health of the supervision relationship'. There are also other skills, such as support and confrontation (Marshall and Confer, 1980), which are necessary in the challenge of supervisees. When good supervision has occurred the supervisee leaves feeling challenged and supported.

Qualities needed by the supervisor include courage, sense of humour, sense of timing, capacity for intimacy and openness to self-inspection (Loganbill, Harding and Delworth, 1982). Courage is needed to confront when necessary and to deal with difficult issues. A sense of humour is useful to relieve tension and to keep fun in the supervision. It is important for the supervisor to know when to intervene and when to overlook certain things. As was stated earlier, clinical supervision occurs within in a relationship so supervisors need to have the capacity for intimacy if they are to make the most of the relationship. Openness to self-inspection needs to be a constant with supervisors if they are to ensure that supervision is used appropriately, rather than to boost their own egos. Finally, a supervisor also needs confidence and professional assurance (Bradley, 1989), as someone who lacks these qualities will be unable to facilitate the professional growth and development of his/her supervisees.

Prospective supervisors must have training and experience within the field in which they plan to supervise. Supervision training must include theoretical information regarding the nature and function of supervision as well as responsibilities of the supervisor. Figure 8.2 identifies the responsibilities of the supervisor.

- Ensuring a safe space for supervisees to lay out practice issues in their own way
- Helping supervisees to explore and clarify thinking, feeling and fantasies that underline their practice
- Sharing information and skills appropriately
- Challenging practice that the supervisor sees as unethical, unwise or incompetent
- Challenging personal and professional blind spots

Figure 8.2 Responsibilities of the supervisor (Hawkins and Shohet, 1989)

Supervision training is not complete without skills training in supervision. This will include the opportunity to practise different aspects of supervising and to receive feedback about one's practice. Some of the skills that will be rehearsed include contracting, setting up supervision, evaluating supervision, techniques of supervision, and so on.

One approach that can be incorporated into training for clinical supervision is coaching, as the interpersonal skills required for effective coaching are similar to those for clinical supervision. Coaching is a familiar concept in sport and athletics, where a skilled coach offers analysis and advice to help a sportsperson or athlete to improve his/her performance. The term is also used in education, where it implies the offering of additional support and tutoring to help a pupil or student to prepare for examinations. Coaching can also be used as a management strategy for improving staff performance at work, and it is in this context that its relevance to clinical supervision becomes apparent.

Some NHS trusts are using a self-study guide called the Coaching Toolkit Programme as part of the preparation for clinical supervision. The Toolkit defines coaching as 'a person-to-person process which helps individuals to come to their own conclusions about the best way to achieve improved performance at work' (South and West Development Forum, 1996). This definition emphasizes the empowerment aspect of coaching: the onus is on the individual to decide how s/he will achieve improved performance. Within an organization, anyone can be a coach to anyone else, provided they have appropriate expertise and experience, and coaching is commonly used to help individuals to acquire new skills, take on new roles, apply learning gained from attendance at courses or study-days, and as part of annual individual performance review.

The key skills identified for coaching are fundamental skills that underpin any interpersonal encounter, including counselling and clinical supervision, and these are listed in Figure 8.3.

- Developing rapport and trust
- Listening
- Summarizing and reflecting
- Self-disclosure
- Questioning
- Giving feedback
- Using silence

Figure 8.3 Coaching skills

The Coaching Toolkit uses a five-stage model with the acronym COACH to help make the coaching session more effective.

- **Circumstance**: In this first stage the coach and the individual attempt to get an overall picture of the current issue for the coaching session.
- **Objective**: The coach helps the individual to formulate the objectives s/he wishes to achieve.
- **Alternatives**: In this stage the range of possible options and alternatives are discussed.
- **Choice**: During this stage, both parties come to a decision about which alternative is most appropriate, given all the factors.
- **Hand-over**: This final stage is about how the choice is to be implemented and the support required to do this.

While the Coaching Toolkit may be a useful training vehicle for clinical supervision, the model needs to be interpreted with flexibility when discussing more contentious issues or ethical dilemmas, and also when working with more experienced staff.

The supervisee

There has been some concern expressed in the nursing literature that those taking on the role of the supervisor should be prepared for that role. This is very important; however, of equal importance is the preparation of the supervisee. Although the nursing literature on this aspect is sparse, Inskipp and Proctor (1993) have written about this in relation to counselling supervision and much of the material is relevant to nursing. It is crucial to train supervisees in how to use supervision prior to implementing any supervision scheme in nursing, midwifery or health visiting. Supervisees may or may not be free to choose their clinical supervisor, depending upon local policy. If a choice is allowed, the supervisee needs to consider the following.

- Is it important to me that my supervisor should be a practitioner from my own specialism?

- Do I prefer a colleague to supervise me or someone from a different department?
- Am I likely to have an open and honest relationship with the supervisor I choose?

The concept of reflection is a key feature of supervision. Many nurses, midwives and health visitors are now familiar with this term, particularly those trained under the Project 2000 scheme. The process of reflection has a number of stages, description of the experience followed by analysis and evaluation (Reid, 1993). Reflection on practice can be seen as a sort of self-supervision that can be used to prepare oneself for supervision with a designated supervisor. Of course, to engage in self-supervision through reflection one must be willing to examine one's strengths and weaknesses. It is also helpful to write things down if one is carrying out this process on one's own.

Recording information is also useful when it comes to taking issues to supervision. Keeping a journal for recording one's reflections is not easy for many practitioners, who are too busy to find extra time for this activity. One way around this is to use the journal for critical incidences only, although the problem with this approach is that many of us will go for long periods without anything we consider critical. A weekly entry could solve this problem as we would then be forced to set aside a time each week when we would reflect on the week's work. Examples of the issues that could be recorded in the journal and subsequently taken to supervision if one needed further help are anxieties about one's work, problems with clients, problems with colleagues, ethical issues, practice/theory issues, research application, etc. It is essential to consider confidentiality and how to ensure it if one keeps a journal. Regardless of whether or not one keeps a reflective journal or not one still has to prepare oneself for supervision in order to get the most out of it.

TYPES OF CLINICAL SUPERVISION

The forms of supervision that a practitioner engages in might be determined by the organization rather than the individual. There are two major categories of supervision, one-to-one and group. These categories can be further broken down into various forms of supervision, which will be examined below.

One-to-one supervision

The most popular form of one-to-one supervision is called individual supervision. Here there is an experienced practitioner who takes the role of the supervisor and a less experienced one who takes the role of supervisee.

This form of supervision 'is still considered the cornerstone of professional development' (Bernard and Goodyear, 1992). It is therefore not surprising that in all five case studies documented in the Kohner Report (1994), this form of supervision was used. As a profession still new to clinical supervision this is probably the best way to start, as this form of supervision is in many ways less complex than some of the others. It also has the advantage of offering more privacy, a higher degree of confidentiality, potentially more time for each supervisee to present their work and gives the supervisor a better overview of the supervisee's work. It is, however, expensive in terms of time, money and personnel, particularly if the supervisor comes from outside the organization.

Group supervision

There are two forms of group supervision, that which has a designated supervisor for the group and that which has peers supervising each other. Each of these forms will be discussed below.

Group supervision with an identified supervisor

In defining this form of supervision, Inskipp and Proctor (1995) said it was:

> a working alliance between a supervisor and several supervisees in which each supervisee can regularly offer an account or recording of his/her work, reflect on it and receive feedback and where appropriate guidance from his/her supervisor and colleagues.

Approaches to using this form of supervision will differ according to the supervisor; some supervisors might supervise individuals within the group while others watch and have a sort of vicarious learning; other supervisors might prefer a more participative approach. One example of getting all the supervisees to be actively involved in the supervision is to give each supervisee a particular issue to concentrate on during the presentation. These could include things such as the client who is being presented, the presenter's relationship with the client s/he is presenting, the interventions used with the client, what is happening within the supervision, etc. A range of other approaches to supervising groups are discussed in Inskipp and Proctor,1995.

The advantages of group supervision are many and include exposing supervisees to alternative modes of helping, enabling them to give and solicit appropriate feedback, aiding in the appreciation of the universality of their concerns (Bradley, 1989), providing a supportive atmosphere for supervisees to share their anxieties (Hawkins and Shohet, 1989) and giving supervisees a broader context in which to judge themselves (Bernard and Goodyear, 1992). Group supervision is economical in terms of time and resources. This is an important consideration in nursing where we have so little time and so few trained supervisors. However, it does not seem to be that popular and in the five case studies referred to in the Kohner Report (1994), only one used group supervision as the primary form of supervision. One reason for this could be that group supervision is a much more complex process than individual supervision and requires skills in group facilitation as well as supervision. There is also the potential problem of the group process being destructive. A disproportionate amount of time could be spent sorting out group process with not enough time left for the content of supervision.

Peer group supervision

Peer supervision or co-supervision is another form of one-to-one supervision where practitioners take turn in supervising each other, e.g. during the first half an hour of the supervision one takes the role as supervisor and the other supervisee; the roles are then reversed for the second half hour. Peer supervision is a formal arrangement in which '[a]ny dis-empowering aspects of supervision as provided by an "expert" are minimised' (Feltham and Dryden, 1994).

Participants having this form of supervision should not have any serious skills deficits and should be experienced in their field as well as having some experience of being supervised by a qualified supervisor.

Peer group supervision has the attraction of a flattened structure, and is economical. It can, however, be rather difficult to run successfully and is best conducted by practitioners who have had experience in supervision. There is also the real possibility of consensus collusion, in which peer group members avoid voicing any criticism or concerns, opting instead to praise colleagues on the reciprocal basis of 'aren't we all wonderful!'.

METHODS AND TECHNIQUES USED IN CLINICAL SUPERVISION

Irrespective of the form of supervision one uses, the method chosen will depend on the supervisees, their learning goals, the resources available to the supervisor and the supervisor's own skills.

Rationale for choice of method

In writing about counselling and psychotherapy supervision Borders and Leddick (1987) give a rationale for choice of method that is applicable to supervision in nursing and health visiting.

The supervisee's learning goals

When setting up supervision it is important to clarify what the supervisee wants to get from supervision. This does not stop a unit from specifying in broad terms how they see supervision and the goals it should achieve. Within that broad frame there should also be space for individuals to specify their own goals, which could be long-term and short-term. Indeed, this is essential, not just for deciding on the method/technique of supervision to be used but also for the evaluation of supervision.

Once the supervisee's goals have been identified then a suitable method of supervision can be chosen to facilitate the attainment of that goal. For example, if the goal is to develop competence in the area of breaking bad news to relatives, the supervisor might want to use such techniques as critical incident analysis or role-play.

The supervisee's experience/level of development

Holloway and Acker, quoted in Holloway, 1995, identified five primary functions of the supervisor:

- monitoring and evaluating
- instructing and advising
- modelling
- consulting
- supporting and sharing.

The amount of time spent on any of these functions will be influenced by the supervisee's experience. For example, with a newly qualified staff nurse more time might be spent on the first three, while for an experienced practitioner more time might be spent on the latter two functions.

The supervisee's learning style

It is inevitable that supervisees will find certain techniques more conducive to their own learning style. For example, an activist who enjoys the here-and-now might find methods such as role-playing and other activity-based forms of supervision more useful than a reflector who prefers to stand back and observe a situation from all angles before doing anything. The reflector might prefer to be given an article to read and reflect on, then discuss in the next supervision session (see Honey, 1982, for further discussion of learning styles).

The supervisor's goals for the supervisee

In addition to what the supervisee identifies as his/her learning goals the supervisor might also have other goals for the supervisee, e.g. working together to identify blind spots.

The supervisor's own learning goals

Supervisors are also learners, who must work to improve their skills and knowledge if they are to keep up to date and effective. This is particularly relevant to nursing, where clinical supervision is still quite new. The supervisor's learning goals may involve practising new techniques s/he wants to develop and this will influence the techniques s/he uses in supervision.

The theoretical orientation of the supervisor

This reason is the only one that is not relevant to nursing. It is useful to note, however, that the supervisor's beliefs about supervision will influence the methods used in supervision. For example, if the belief is that supervision should be purely content-focused then methods involving the process of supervision will not be used.

Methods and techniques available

Having identified the factors that affect the choice of methods/techniques it is now appropriate to look at some of the methods/techniques available.

- **Reflective journal**: This is a written record of the supervisee's reflections on incidents that have occurred in his/her practice. The supervisee might choose to use information from this journal as the basis for supervision.
- **Critical incident analysis**: The supervisee brings along a critical incident s/he wants to reflect on. This is similar to the use of reflective journals, except that the self-supervision used through reflection might not have occurred prior to supervision.
- **Role-play/role-reversal**: This can be used to explore role behaviour in the work situation as well as helping resolve problems when the supervisee feels stuck and wants to find alternative ways forward. In role reversal the supervisee takes the role of the other party involved in the problem; this can give valuable insights into the feelings of another.
- **Modelling**: Here the supervisor shows the supervisee 'how it is done'. For example, if a nurse has problems in setting limits/boundaries for clients the supervisor might model limit setting for him/her in the way s/he sets limits for the supervisee's presentation.
- **Teaching**: This involves providing theoretical inputs at appropriate points during the supervision in order to fill certain gaps in the supervisee's knowledge, e.g. sharing some recent research that might affect the care of the client who is being presented.
- **Suggested reading**: Some supervisees prefer reading material they can take away to read and absorb at their own pace.
- **Sculpting**: This technique can be used in group supervision and can be used with good effect in situations where supervisees might be working with groups or families. For example, a health visitor who is having problems dealing with a family could be asked to position the family members as she sees them. (Members of the supervision group could be used for the various family members.) The supervisor could also ask the health visitor presenting the case to fit him/herself into the sculpture. Questions might then be addressed to the various members in the sculpture to ascertain the thoughts and feelings they are having as it relates to their positioning. This sort of sculpting/positioning could give valuable insights into the family.

- **Parallel process**: Often what is happening in the supervision session replicates what happened in the nurse/client relationship, so if the supervisor attends to the process of the here-and-now relationship of the supervision she might help the supervisee to see the parallels and to understand what is happening within that relationship with the client.

IMPLEMENTING CLINICAL SUPERVISION

The working relationship

One of the most important aspects of clinical supervision is the relationship between supervisors and supervisees. Mutual trust is required, and this could take some time to develop, particularly if there was no choice in the selection of the supervisor.

Many supervisees are not given a choice of supervisor so it is important to think of ways of dealing with this situation. One way of doing this is for the supervisor to use some of the time in the first session to look at what it is like for the supervisee working with a supervisor s/he did not choose. The supervisor could also share his/her concerns about the matter before looking at ways in which they can both get the best out of their times together.

Bringing the matter out in the open can be a good way of clearing the air and facilitating a more open relationship that is likely to lead to trust. Other factors that might help in the trust-building are the establishment of norms and boundaries and the limits of confidentiality.

In their work with supervisees, supervisors should adopt a non-judgemental stance, because if supervisees feel judged they will not be willing to share areas of their work that they suspect might be inefficient, nor will they be open to learning from the supervisor (Inskipp and Proctor, 1993). The relationship between the supervisor and supervisee is one that needs constant attention if it is to be supportive, challenging and produce growth. It is quite easy for the relationship to be too comfortable and when it is, both clients and practitioners are likely suffer in some way. Similarly, the relationship can become too uncomfortable for any useful work to take place.

Implementing one-to-one supervision

A supervision contract is a useful way of clarifying the working agreement, as well as making for an easier relationship, since everyone knows where they stand. Figure 8.4 shows the components normally included in a supervision contract.

Arranging the time and place of supervision meetings may seem straightforward, but in practice there can be snags. Offices are rarely appropriate for clinical supervision, as constant disturbance can be expected from telephones and visitors. Cowes and Wilkes (1998) report that 'all members wanted to get away

- Practical arrangements, i.e. time, place, frequency and length of meetings
- Record-keeping arrangements
- What will happen in the case of missed sessions
- Confidentiality
- What will happen in the case of incompetent practice
- What communication if any there will be between the supervisor and the supervisee's manager
- What access (if any) the supervisee will have to the supervisor between sessions

Figure 8.4 Elements of a supervision contract

from their immediate working environment in order that privacy could be ensured and distractions minimised'. Difficulty may be experienced in finding a suitably private room that is not already booked, particularly if several clinical supervision meetings are taking place on the same day. Over-running of a previous meeting is a common occurrence, resulting in erosion of the time available for the next meeting; 1 hour is a reasonable time allocation but timing will vary depending on local circumstances. The problem of room bookings is further compounded where supervision for practice nurses and health visitors takes place in rooms in GP surgeries, because the use of such rooms may be chargeable and this will impact on the overall resource provision for clinical supervision.

Given that both parties to clinical supervision are busy practitioners, it is likely that one or both will arrive late from time to time. When negotiating the supervision contract, it is useful to allow a margin for late arrival; e.g. they might agree to wait up to half an hour for the other to arrive. This margin can help reduce panic reactions, such as driving too fast to get to the meeting on time. The time of day at which the meeting takes place will vary according to local circumstances, but many supervisors and supervisees prefer the end of the day, when patient/client demand may be less. The frequency of meetings varies widely in the literature, ranging from weekly to 3-monthly.

It is important that both supervisor and supervisee keep records of clinical supervision for their personal professional profile as evidence of professional development. While these records are confidential to the individuals concerned, it is also necessary to keep a managerial record of clinical supervision that contains the minimum amount of information required by management, in order to be able to confirm that supervision has occurred and to enable the time to be costed. This information would normally be the names of the supervisor and supervisee, the dates on which supervision took place and the reasons for any cancellation. In cases of litigation by patients or clients, such records can provide evidence of the ongoing professional development of the practitioner involved.

The first meeting between the clinical supervisor and supervisee tends to be the most difficult, since both parties may be unsure about how to proceed. It is helpful if this first meeting focuses on negotiating the supervision contract, as the process of negotiation will itself help to encourage the development of rapport between the two parties. Since the contract contains tangible aspects such as practical arrangements and record-keeping, it provides a less threatening focus for discussion in the initial phase of the meeting when the parties are at their most anxious.

In order to get the most benefit from supervisory meetings, it is helpful if the supervisee can undertake some prior preparation. The example below shows the form such preparation might take.

Context: I am a newly qualified staff nurse working in a neurological unit. I have monthly clinical supervision from the link tutor to the unit. My next supervision session is tomorrow and I have given myself half an hour to prepare for it.

Stages in the preparation

Stage 1: (Reflect on what has happened at work since my last supervision.) I examined my reflective journal and noted the three incidents I had recorded since my last supervision. The first was a record of an incident regarding discharge of a client, the second was an argument with a colleague about my off-duty and the third was a request from a client (Mrs X) not to tell her relatives about her diagnosis.

Stage 2: (Deciding which of the issues is foreground for me.) I decided to use the incident with Mrs X as it was the most recent and I was still uneasy about it.

Stage 3: (Reflect on the incident chosen or remind myself of reflections I had already done.) In reflecting on the incident with Mrs X I asked myself the following questions:

- What did Mrs X actually say to me?
- What did I think was behind her request?
- What did I think were her feelings when she made her request?
- What did I think as I listened to her request?
- What did I feel as I listened to her request?
- How did I respond?
- How else could I have responded?
- What issues are still outstanding for me?

Stage 4: (Identifying what I want from supervision.) From my reflection on the incident I identified the following things that I wanted from supervision:

1. to explore alternative ways of responding to the situation;
2. to examine why the incident made me feel so uneasy.

This example shows how prior preparation can lead to the clear identification of issues to be raised in the clinical supervision meeting, and it is interesting to note that the two points identified include both formative and restorative elements. Some difficulty may be experienced by supervisors whose role involves them in conducting individual performance reviews on a regular basis. The focus of IPR is very much on the measuring of outcomes, and supervisors may find it difficult to adapt this directive style to fit clinical supervision. In this case, training must be provided to help them to adopt a more appropriate interactive style.

Implementing group supervision

To get the most out of group supervision there are certain factors that should be considered.

The size and composition of the group

The size of the group should range from three to seven people. The larger the group, the less time each individual has to present and conversely the more space each individual will have to hide. If the group is too small then issues such as absences and dropout become more of a problem as there might not be enough people left to operate as a group.

The second issue to consider is who will make up the group. It could be that the group is made up of people from the same team. This arrangement can be advantageous in that all are familiar with the client group, the context and each other. There are, however, disadvantages, such as having to deal with ongoing difficult group dynamics that have no direct relation to the supervision but influence it. Another possible problem of having staff from the same team is the mix of experience: Chaiklin and Manson (1983) argue that in mixed groups there is a tendency for experienced supervisees to lose out.

An alternative to supervising staff in work teams would be to supervise staff of a similar grade and from a similar clinical area, e.g. F-grade staff nurses working in high-dependency areas. One of the advantages of this approach is the freshness of perspective that supervisees bring to the work. Fear of issues discussed in the supervision being taken back to one's place of work is also lessened. Responsibility for the composition of the group may rest with the clinical manager, the supervisor or the supervisee. All these options have advantages and disadvantages.

Ultimately, the supervisor needs to be happy with the composition of the group, otherwise this could lead to unnecessary difficulties.

Who will supervise the group?

A clinical supervisor working with groups should have training as a supervisor and possess skills in group facilitation. Likely people for this role might be link tutors, specialist nurses or clinical managers. It may be useful for clinical managers from neighbouring hospitals to have a reciprocal arrangement where they supervise each other's staff.

How will the group work?

Once the composition of the group has been decided the supervisor meets with the group to discuss how they will work together as a group. One of the first things that must be discussed in the group is the supervisees' understanding and expectation of supervision. This is crucial to setting the scene, as views regarding supervision differ and if the group is to work together in a satisfactory way there must be shared understanding. Mismatch of expectations can also play havoc with a group. The supervisee's past experience of supervision may also influence the supervision process so it is useful to discuss this and work through any unfinished business.

Early in the supervision the supervisor needs to find out how each supervisee learns best. The reason for this is that the supervisor could then choose methods/techniques of supervision that will meet the needs of the supervisees' learning styles. Linked to this should be a discussion regarding the structure of the supervision group, as structure helps to reduce anxiety. The structure should allow for some degree of flexibility so as not to stifle spontaneity. The supervision contract should also be discussed at this time and each supervisee should identify what s/he wants to get from supervision. It is important for each supervisee to know what the others want because it is only then that they can work together to help each other to achieve their goals.

Ground rules need to be established at the initial stage of the group. This should include how poor professional practice will be dealt with and the limits to confidentiality. For example, is the supervisor required to give management a report on the supervision and if so what should be the content of that report and will the supervisee have a say in the writing of it? Other ground rules might concern time-keeping, presentation, etc. In addition to the discussions and negotiations within the group, the supervisor needs to clarify certain things for him/herself. These include how s/he will go about encouraging supervisees to take risks within the group. Risk-taking is essential for growth and development but unless supervisees feel safe they will not risk exposing their most vulnerable areas of work. This could be a problem, as often this is just the sort of work they should be taking to supervision. Supervisors need to examine how they are going to foster group cohesion and participation from all their supervisees.

Implementing peer group supervision

Successful peer supervision, like any other form of supervision, requires careful preparation. Therefore, before embarking on peer supervision, participants should ask themselves the following questions.

- Have I done any reading on peer supervision?
- Am I clear about what is involved?
- Who do I want as my peer in this supervisory relationship?
- Is our attitude to each other that of cooperation or competition?

- Do we share similar value systems?
- What makes me think I can work with this person?
- Where will we meet? Will this place be free of interruptions?
- How frequently will we meet and how long will each session last?
- Will the sessions be taped and if so how will the tape be used?
- Is there time set aside to process each session?
- How frequently will we evaluate the supervision process as a whole?

These questions should help to clarify whether or not peer supervision is likely to be appropriate in any given case.

Who should be in the group?

Often peer groups are made up of friends and while this is helpful in making supervisees comfortable it can get too cosy and may break down into social chitchat. One way to prevent this is to set up the group so that there is a time for socializing before the group starts. It might even be useful to nominate different members from week to week to manage the time boundary.

How large will the group be?

Schreiber and Frank (1983) suggested that a peer group should have at least seven members. Groups larger than seven are not recommended, as it makes for rather complex group dynamics, and the larger the group the less space there is for supervisees to present. We do, however, appreciate these writers' concern about dropouts and absences in smaller groups. There are ways of dealing with this difficulty and these matters should be discussed early in the life of the group.

How to format the group?

It is often useful for members of a peer group to have roles, as this helps to structure the process. Marks and Hixon (1986) suggested the need for a process observer whose role it is to give feedback about the process of supervision. This person would have no other role in the group during that session. Other roles might be presenters or supervisor. These roles can be rotated from meeting to meeting.

What ground rules should the group have?

This is an important issue for any supervision group but is even more so in peer supervision where there is no designated leader/supervisor.

How will the supervision be evaluated and how often?

A format for evaluation needs to be agreed as well as setting evaluation dates.

MANAGEMENT ISSUES IN CLINICAL SUPERVISION

The advent of clinical supervision, focusing as it does on the professional practice of individuals, may be regarded with scepticism or suspicion by some participants.

Prospective supervisors may see it as an unnecessary, time-consuming activity that diverts resources from direct patient/client care. Supervisees may be suspicious of the motives of managers in introducing clinical supervision, seeing it as a covert means of disciplining staff for inadequate practice. The relative lack of opportunities for promotion in the health-care sector and the widespread use of short-term contracts for staff can make for a competitive climate in which trust is not readily apparent. Staff may consider it naive to openly and honestly disclose important aspects of their professional practice to a clinical supervisor, particularly if they feel that such disclosure might adversely affect their future employment prospects. It is also possible that some models of clinical supervision may give staff the impression that it is a counselling intervention or, at worst, some kind of amateur psychotherapy. Organizations planning to introduce clinical supervision need to make strenuous efforts to overcome these reservations, otherwise the process of clinical supervision will become a mere charade. McCallion and Baxter (1995) state that:

> whether or not staff are resistant to the initiative depends upon the way that clinical supervision is presented to practitioners and the way it is implemented. Practitioners should be fully involved in the implementation and encouraged to take ownership of it in their area.

Figure 8.5 identifies a range of factors that organizations need to consider when planning to introduce clinical supervision.

A. Fowler, 1996
- Target group of staff
- Purpose of supervision for that group
- Criteria for appointment as clinical supervisor
- Nature of the supervisory relationship
- Time involvement
- Need for an agreement or contract

B. McCallion and Baxter, 1995
- Choosing a model of supervision
- Identifying and training the supervisors and supervisees
- Staff resistance
- Time element
- Cost implications
- Maintenance of records
- Evaluation and audit

Figure 8.5 Factors to be considered when planning to introduce clinical supervision

Implementation can be facilitated by the appointment of a lead individual whose responsibility is to establish clinical supervision within the organization, including training and monitoring.

Each organization will need to draw up a policy statement on clinical supervision that is flexible enough to meet local requirements, and make this available to all staff so that they know exactly the parameters in which the supervision will operate. Figure 8.6 shows the aspects normally included in a policy statement on clinical supervision.

- A clear definition of clinical supervision which distinguishes it from managerial concepts such as individual performance review
- The philosophy and rationale for the introduction of clinical supervision, including the aims and perceived benefits to patient/client care, to individual practitioners and to the organization
- The nature of confidentiality in clinical supervision, including instances where confidentiality may be breached
- Guidelines on which professionals should supervise others – it is commonly found that organizations suggest that nurses supervise colleagues of the same grade as themselves, and all grades below
- Guidelines on how supervisors are chosen or allocated, and how supervisees may change their supervisor
- Guidelines on the frequency of supervision and time allowance for each meeting
- Guidelines on the reflective process for supervisees
- Details of the training that is available for supervisors

Figure 8.6 Components of a policy statement on clinical supervision

Unforeseen difficulties arising from clinical supervision my have an unexpected impact on practice. For example, there may be ethical conflicts in cases where a supervisee gains promotion and becomes the line manager of his/her clinical supervisor, given that issues discussed during clinical supervision are not normally disclosed to the line manager. The following real-life example also illustrates an unexpected difficulty.

A practitioner happens to share an office with a managerial colleague who acts as line manager to a number of staff. As part of her role, the practitioner would normally discuss issues concerning these members of staff with their line manager, but she has recently taken on the role of clinical supervisor to one of these members of staff. Since commencing supervision, she is reluctant to discuss the staff member who is her supervisee with the line manager, because she is afraid that she might inadvertently disclose something confidential from a supervisory meeting.

EVALUATION OF SUPERVISION

There are still huge gaps in the profession's awareness of the effectiveness of clinical supervision in nursing, and evaluation is one of the means of bridging that gap.

Evaluation is about making judgements and one of the judgements we need to make is about the effectiveness of supervision. This leads to the question of how effectiveness is defined, and who makes that decision. Effectiveness has to do with whether or not the supervision is achieving the aims for which it was implemented. To gain this sort of information we need feedback from clients and their relatives, managers, supervisors and supervisees. In evaluating the supervision, supervisors and supervisees will need to examine their working relationship, the content of the supervision session and the resources available. It is important not just to get feedback from each other but to engage in our own self-evaluation.

Supervisees might want to consider how far they are meeting their supervision goals and hindering or helping them.

Supervisors might want to consider how they are doing at balancing the tasks of supervision and how sensitive they are to the learning styles of their supervisees.

Butterworth, Bishop and Carson (1996) suggest using the elements of clinical supervision as defined by Proctor (1991) as the basis of an evaluation strategy. In relation to the formative or educational element, evaluation could be carried out by analysis of videotape or audiotape recordings of supervision, and by analysis of observation notes. The restorative element could be evaluated using a range of instruments to survey staff well-being and stress, and for the normative element they suggest that a range of existing data could be used such as clinical audit data, sickness/absence rates, number of patient complaints, etc.

REFERENCES

Armitage, P. and Burnard, P. (1991) Mentors or preceptors? Narrowing the theory-practice gap. *Nurse Education Today*, **11**, 225–229.

Atherton, J. (1986) *Professional Supervision in Group Care: A Contract Based Approach*, Tavistock, London.

Bernard, J. and Goodyear, R. (1992) *Fundamentals of Clinical Supervision*, Allyn & Bacon, London.

Bishop, V. (1994) Clinical supervision for an accountable profession. *Nursing Times*, **90**(39).

Borders, L. and Leddick, G. (1987) *Handbook of Counseling Supervision*, Association for Counselor Education and Supervision, Alexandria, VA.

Bradley, L. (1989) *Counselor Supervision: Principles, Process and Practice*, Accelerated Development, Muncie, IN.

Butterworth, T., Bishop, B. and Carson, J. (1996) First steps towards evaluating clinical supervision in nursing and health visiting: 1. Theory, policy and practice development. a review. *Journal of Clinical Nursing*, **5**, 127–132.

Chaiklin, H. and Manson, C. (1983) Peer consultation in social work. *Clinical Supervisor*, **1**, 24–34.

Cowes, F. and Wilkes, C. (1998) Clinical supervision for specialist nurses. *Professional Nurse*, **13**(5).

Davies, P. (1993) Value yourself. *Nursing Times*, **89**(4).

Department of Health (1993) *Vision for the Future*, HMSO, London.

ENB (1993) *Regulations and Guidelines for the Approval of Institutions and Courses*, English National Board for Nursing, Midwifery and Health Visiting, London.

Faugier, J. and Butterworth, T. (1994) *Clinical Supervision: A Positional Paper*, School of Nursing, University of Manchester, Manchester.

Feltham, C. and Dryden, W. (1994) *Developing Counsellor Supervision*, Sage, London.

Fisher, M. (1996) Using reflective practice in clinical supervision. *Professional Nurse*, **11**(7).

Fowler, J. (1996) How to use models of clinical supervision in practice. *Nursing Standard*, **10**(29).

Hawkins, P. and Shohet, R. (1989) *Supervision in the Helping Professions*, Open University Press, Milton Keynes.

Holloway, E. (1995) *Clinical Supervision: A Systems Approach*, Sage, London.

Honey, P. (1982) *The Manual of Learning Styles*, Honey & Mumford, Maidenhead.

Inskipp, F. and Proctor, B. (1993) *Making the Most of Supervision*, Cascade, London.

Inskipp, F. and Proctor, B. (1995) *Becoming a Supervisor*, Cascade, London.

Kohner, N. (1994) *Clinical Supervision in Practice*, King's Fund, London.

Loganbill, C., Harding, E. and Delworth, U. (1982) Supervision: a conceptual model. *Counseling Psychologist*, **10**, 3–42.

Marks, J. and Hixon, D. (1986) Training agency staff through peer supervision. *Social Casework*, **67**, 418–423.

Marshall, W. and Confer, W. (1980) Psychotherapy supervision: supervisees' perspective, in *Psychotherapy Supervision: Theory, Research and Practice*, (ed. A. K. Hess), John Wiley, New York, pp. 92–100.

McCallion, H. and Baxter, T. (1995) Clinical supervision: take it from the top. *Nursing Management*, **1**(9).

McGibbon, G. (1996) Clinical supervision for expanded practice in ENT. *Professional Nurse*, **12**(2).

Proctor, B. (1991) Supervision: a co-operative exercise in accountability, in *Enabling and Ensuring Supervision in Practice*, (eds M. Markem and M. Payne), National Youth Bureau and Council for Education and Training in Youth and Community Work, Leicester, pp. 21–23.

Quinn, F. M. (1995) *The Principles and Practice of Nurse Education*, 3rd edn, Stanley Thornes, Cheltenham.

Reid, B. (1993) But we are doing it already: exploring response to the concept of reflective practice in order to improve its facilitation. *Nurse Education Today*, **13**, 305–309.

Schreiber, P. and Frank, E. (1983) The use of supervision in groups by social work clinicians. *Clinical Supervisor*, **1**(1), 29–36.

South and West Development Forum (1996) *The Coaching Toolkit Programme*, Foreward, Cheshire.

Swain, G. (1995) *Clinical Supervision: The Principles and Process*, Health Visitors Association, London.

UKCC (1992) *Code of Professional Conduct*, United Kingdom Central Council for Nursing, Midwifery and Health Visiting, London.

UKCC (1996a) *Position Statement on Clinical Supervision for Nursing and Health Visiting*, United Kingdom Central Council for Nursing, Midwifery and Health Visiting, London.

UKCC (1996b) *Issues Arising from Professional Conduct Complaints*, United Kingdom Central Council for Nursing, Midwifery and Health Visiting, London.

9

The power of the professional profile

Liz Redfern

INTRODUCTION

Using a profile to help you keep a record of your professional life and development is not difficult, and is certainly within the capability of all nurses, midwives and health visitors. Despite this, it could be argued that, out of all the PREPP proposals, the requirement to maintain a personal professional profile has caused the most anxiety and concern. This is probably because we are unsure of what is expected.

This chapter will address some of the background on why nurses are now expected to use profiles, and in an easy and accessible way show you how to get started and maintain a profile to meet United Kingdom Central Council (UKCC) requirements. In doing that the chapter will also identify and discuss the many issues that have been raised within the profession because of the introduction of profiles, such as confidentiality and ownership.

Common concerns and questions

Any forum where profiles are being discussed tends to involve similar questions being asked by the participants. I thought it might be useful at this point in the chapter to introduce some of those common questions and explain the typical answers.

I have heard the word profile and portfolio used interchangeably; is there a difference?

The products on sale to nurses use different names to describe essentially the same thing. Even the statutory bodies have chosen to go different ways with their terminology, with the UKCC naming it a personal professional profile and the English National Board (ENB) naming theirs a professional portfolio. A brief look at the literature shows that variation too. Some of the definitions are given below.

- Redman (1994): 'a portfolio is simply a tangible record of what someone has done'; he does not bother to make a distinction between a profile and a portfolio.
- Brown (1992) does. She defines the term personal portfolio as:

    a private collection of evidence which demonstrates the continuing acqui-
    sition of skills, knowledge, attitudes, understanding and achievement. It
    is both retrospective and prospective, as well as reflecting the current
    stage of development of the individual.

    She goes on to define a profile as 'a collection of evidence which is selected from the personal portfolio for a particular purpose and for the attention of a particular audience'.

- Hull and Redfern (1996) offer the following definitions: *Portfolio*: a private collection of a wide range of evidence and items of interest to you – it might contain personal and professional items. *Profile*: is a selection of specific evidence for a specific purpose to present to a specific audience (for example, for the UKCC requirements).

It is difficult to know why and how this differing use of the terms has arisen, and to some extent it doesn't matter. Having identified that confusion exists alerts us to the fact that it is important to find out how someone is using the term so that you are able to share their perceptions before jumping to conclusions.

Generally speaking, whatever word is used to describe it there are characteristics that are common to a profile and a portfolio. They usually:

- value experience as a source of learning;
- encourage reflective practice;
- provide a storehouse for information about and evidence of experience, learning and achievements;
- encourage personal and professional development.

Do I need to buy a ready-made profile or can I make my own?

The straight answer to this is no, you do not need to buy a ready-made profile to meet UKCC requirements. However, you may find that to complete certain educational programmes you may have to use a particular profile, which is sold to you as part of the registration fee.

The key thing about keeping a profile is that you have to organize its contents in such a way that you can find them again. It is a bit like having a personal filing cabinet of information about your professional life and at times you will need go to a file and draw out a particular piece of paper. This means having it organized and labelled in such a way that you can reliably find things again once you have filed them away. There are many different approaches to filing information away and you should use a system that means something to you.

The UKCC recognize that there are many different types of profile available and they have not endorsed any particular one. This quite rightly leaves the decision to you.

The ready-made profiles have been designed by others and they use their preferred order for the sections. Their order may not be yours, and you need to have a good look at one before buying to make sure you feel comfortable with the layout. Also, remember that you can change the sections around and add to them in a way that makes sense to you. The advantage of buying a ready-made profile is that the publishers are likely to have drawn on the expertise of people with an insight into the philosophy behind profiling and you are getting that expertise in the price you pay.

For busy professionals a ready-made profile also gives you the advantage of not having to think about how to build up and organize your own profile from scratch. At a profile workshop recently a staff nurse said to me, 'I am having enough problems trying to get started on my profile, let alone make my own. I'm really pleased I can buy one off the shelf'. A good point.

Remember, many of the ready-made profiles were produced before the UKCC finalized their thoughts about profiles, so they do not necessarily follow the UKCC's intentions. The contents of these profiles often take you beyond the UKCC requirements. A recent innovation has been the introduction of electronic versions of profiles and portfolios. These are ideal for someone who is computer-literate and would prefer to use this medium to store and update his/her personal professional profile. Hopefully in the near future interactive software could be developed, either on disc or through CD-ROM technology, not only to help people store information but to take them through exercises to help them understand their professional practice and development needs much more clearly.

Some trusts have had profiles designed for their staff to use and have issued them free of charge to all nursing employees. This is very helpful and can illustrate how supportive employers intend to be in helping their nursing staff achieve the UKCC requirements. However, it often leads to the next question.

Who owns my profile?

Writing about yourself and your professional practice in your profile will probably mean you are including confidential information that you would not wish anyone else to read. Your profile is just that, **your** profile, and no one can see it without your permission. It is advisable not to document any information that could identify patients, clients or colleagues so you are not breaching confidentiality. The way you organize the information in your profile is important.

The UKCC in their publication *PREP and YOU* (1997) state:

Your profile is your personal document. It does not belong to the UKCC or your employer and its contents are private and confidential to you. Your employer or manager does not have the right to look at it.

If you are keeping a profile for other than UKCC purposes you should establish at the beginning with the person or organization that has asked you to keep one what the purpose of the profile is. For example, universities often ask you to prepare a profile as part of an application for a programme of study. This may be to your advantage as it can be used to assess whether you will be allowed to enter the programme without the expected entry qualification. However, you still need to know who will want to see which parts of the profile and what they are going to do with it. Will they show it to other people and for what reason? Will they copy it? How will they store it while it is in their possession? You have a right to know the answers to these questions and anyone asking you to keep a profile should have thought through the issues raised by the questions and have reasonable answers for you.

There have been some instances where, because a trust has supplied staff with a profile, managers believe they have a right to read it from time to time or to use it as part of your annual performance review. A profile can be a very useful source of information within a performance review system, but that information should be extracted by you and adapted as necessary within the review paperwork. Handing over the whole profile in these circumstances is never the right answer.

How do I know what the UKCC wants?

The UKCC issued everyone on the register with a free collection of PREPP Fact Sheets early in 1995. They have also included follow-up articles in *Register*, which is issued quarterly. The Fact Sheets are well written and easy to understand and they outline the main points about all aspects of PREPP. They are a really useful resource to refer to when you feel confused or have forgotten what you need to do. In October 1997, the UKCC issued a new booklet *PREP and YOU*, which supersedes the Fact Sheets. Although the booklet does contain some very useful new information and in many ways replicates the Fact Sheets, the details about what to record in the profile have been taken out. This is unfortunate and means that the new booklet is not as helpful about profiles as the old Fact Sheets. My advice would be to keep your Fact Sheets as useful reference material. The list of what the UKCC expects you to record in your profile is included later in this chapter.

When do I need to start?

Although the introduction of the legislation to implement PREPP occurred in April 1995, it will be implemented over a period of time to allow all registrants to come into the system when their normal registration renewal time is due. For example, my registration renewal date is November 1997 and my reregistration notification will tell me that if I wish to reregister in November 2000 I will need to show that I have been:

- maintaining my professional knowledge and competence by completing the minimum of 5 days updating; and
- recording that activity in my personal profile along with other key personal and professional details.

Everyone will be in the system by 2001. The 3-year lead-in time is not supposed to give you a false sense of security or to encourage you not to bother with profiles and updating now. It does give you the chance to think about what you need to do and work steadily towards the PREPP requirements.

Where have profiles come from and why has nursing decided to use them?

The idea of using profiles and portfolios started in the American higher education system as a way of increasing the number of people, particularly mature students, who could access part-time and full-time programmes of study. In this context profiles were used to show what potential students had learnt from their past experiences. Once the evidence of this learning, which was written up in a profile, had been assessed the student was able to gain credit for that previous learning. This credit then replaced formal entrance qualifications or parts of the programme. This resulted in the student not being expected to repeat learning they had already acquired. The use of profiles in this way now also happens in the UK because of a system called the Credit Accumulation and Transfer Scheme (CATS) and the use of the concept of experiential learning.

The American trend arrived in UK higher education in the early 1980s and by the early 1990s the first references to profiles appeared in the nursing literature. Profiles are now seen as a tool that can be used to develop a habit of lifelong learning, as well as gaining access to programmes of study.

When the UKCC started the Post Registration Education Practice Project they had to find a way of ensuring nurses kept up to date and continued to develop as professionals after their initial qualifying course that enabled them to become registered. The project team rejected the American nursing model of collecting continuing education points largely through attendance at approved study days. This model was criticized for focusing more on the ability to attend and collect points than on identifying clearly what the nurse had learnt from attending and, more importantly, how s/he might have applied that learning into day-to-day practice. The project team decided that a profiling process linked to a flexible approach to achieving a minimum of 5 days updating in every 3-year period would be better. Maintaining a profile matched more closely the values of professional accountability that the UKCC already embodied in its policy statements.

So, as you can see, nursing and the UKCC did not invent the concept of profiling, but they were able to take the best aspects of their use from adult education and apply them to the specific purpose of the continued professional development of nurses and midwives. The PREP Project has had a great influence on how widely profiles are being used in nursing and midwifery. According to Hull and Redfern (1996), other influences have included:

- the National Boards;
- the rise of reflective practice;
- market forces from those publishers selling profiles.

What are the links between the UKCC profile and days of updating?

The UKCC expects you to make an accurate record of all your learning activities in your profile. The updating activity should fall into the five broad categories the UKCC has established. These are:

- patient, client and colleague support (supervision of clinical practice, counselling and leadership);
- care enhancement (standard-setting or new techniques and approaches to care);
- practice development (personal research/study or relevant visits to practice settings);
- reducing risk (health promotion or screening);
- education development (personal research/study or exchange arrangements).

The categories are meant to give great flexibility to the types of activity you choose to get involved in to meet the minimum of 5 days updating. The time factor of 5 days is also meant to be flexible in the way it is used. You need to accumulate 5 days' worth of activity but it does not mean you have to attend five study days that fall into the categories. For example, an activity could be time you use in a library to do personal research and study on a topic relevant to your practice. The important thing is that you can provide evidence in your profile of:

- how much time you spent;
- what you were trying to achieve;
- what you learnt from the activity;
- how you tried to apply that learning to your practice;
- an evaluation of that application.

THE THEORETICAL BASE UNDERPINNING PROFILES

The introduction of profiles into the world of nursing and midwifery has brought with it theories that stem from an educational philosophy about the way adults learn. The two main theories are those associated with experiential learning and reflective practice.

Experiential learning is largely concerned with learning that takes place when you are directly involved with the reality of the situation being studied. We have all experienced hearing about something in a lecture, but it doesn't really make sense or sink in until we have to care for someone with that condition. Bringing the reality of practice to learning makes a real difference.

In more recent times the work of Kolb (1984) has tried to explain how we learn from experience. He argues for a relationship between thinking and experience. He views experiential learning as a cycle involving action and reflection, theory and practice.

The cycle implies that one stage automatically follows another, but in reality not all experiences are transformed into general concepts; all concepts are not analysed; and not all concepts are tested out in the world. According to Sheckley and Keeton (1994), the flow of the stages and how they are used depend upon the person trying to learn from the experience.

So far, then, we have said that experiential learning involves not merely theory but practice, not simply observing but doing. This is one of the reasons why it is seen as a particularly effective approach to professional education. If we really do gain so much quality learning from our life and social situations, we have to acknowledge the importance of our emotions in this process.

So, for example, much of our best learning is often gained from highly emotionally charged experiences such as bereavement, falling in love and divorce.

Reflection is now recognized as an essential component of professional practice, particularly since the publication of Donald Schon's *The Reflective Practitioner* in 1983. Indeed, reflection is viewed by Kolb as an active process that **turns** the experience into learning. An educationalist, David Boud, who is based in Australia, has written extensively on the role of reflection in learning. Boud (Boud, Keogh and Walker, 1985) takes the view that most of us are largely unaware of our internal processes for learning. However, once we become aware and skilled at using them we are likely to become much more effective practitioners. So, for Boud, reflection is simply a generic term for the mental activities we engage in in order for learning to occur.

BENEFITS OF A PROFILE

On the basis of these theories identified above the UKCC believe that your profile has two important functions for you as a professional.

- It will contribute to your professional development by helping you to recognize, understand and value your abilities, strengths, achievements and experience.
- It provides a source of information upon which you can draw at any time, and if required to do so by the UKCC.

The UKCC believe a profile will:

- help you assess your current standards of practice;
- develop your analytical skills;
- enable you to review and evaluate past experience and learning regularly, in order to plan and negotiate your continuing education and career moves;

- provide effective, up-to-date information for use in application forms and interviews when you apply for jobs or courses;
- provide evidence of what you have learned from experience.

MAKING A START

It really does not matter where you start to build your UKCC profile. It needs to start in the place that makes most sense to you and in the area that feels the easiest to achieve. No one expects you to sit down in one go and fill in all the sections at once or that you will be able to reflect on 20 years of nursing experience.

It is probably a good idea to go back to what the UKCC expect you to store in your profile. Once you have looked at the list below, which comes from UKCC Fact Sheet 4, you can decide what looks the easiest or most comfortable to start writing down.

What do the UKCC expect you to record in your profile?

- **Factual information:**
    - Personal/biographical information
    - Professional registerable qualifications
    - Recordable qualifications
    - Other academic qualifications
    - Positions held throughout your career
    - Other activities/positions you hold/have held outside your job
- **Self-appraisal of professional performance:**
    - Your strengths and weaknesses
    - Your achievements
    - Notes from your analysis of significant events
    - Areas in which you want to develop
- **Record of goals and action plans:**
    - Write down your goals, your action plans, a timescale for achieving them and a schedule of dates for reviewing progress.
    - Each time you review your goals, describe and record your progress. If necessary revise goals and action plans.
    - Record the outcomes of your action plans as you achieve them.
- **Record of formal learning:**
    - Study days/seminars, courses and conferences you attend
    - Visits to other units or places of interest and relevance to your work
    - Time spent in the library for, e.g., carrying out a literature search
    For each formal learning experience you will need to describe:
    - its relevance to your professional practice and development;
    - what you hope to achieve from it;
    - your assessment of the outcomes of your activities;

   – the time spent on each event and any follow-up work.
- **Record of your working hours**
   – Record for each 3-year period.

Look at the list: read it through several times. Be aware of which headings seem easy and which make you think 'How will I do that?' (Redfern, 1997). Start with the easy ones and plan to achieve a small step at a time. As you finish each small step you will be building your confidence to do more. A lot of people find the straightforward factual information (such as name; qualifications; jobs you have had) the easiest point to start. It is likely that you will have written them down before on a job application or CV, so you may already have the information recorded in a logical way. If you have, then just transfer it to your profile. All the ready-made profiles have sections already laid out to help you recall the relevant information. The headings above also cover the areas in which the UKCC might request information from you in the future, so I would advise you to document the information corresponding to these headings.

THE PROFILING PROCESS

Building and maintaining a profile is much more than storing factual information about yourself and your career, it is a continuous process. There are three steps to the process, which need to be connected to each other and performed at regular intervals for the rest of your professional life. These steps may seem an over-whelming task at the moment, but in time, like learning any skill, it will become easier and like any other good professional habit. The UKCC identify the three steps as:

1. reviewing your experience to date;
2. self-appraisal;
3. setting goals and action plans.

Step 1: Reviewing your experience to date

The UKCC are only expecting you to look in detail at the last 3 years, but there may be experiences from further back in your career that are significant to you for some reason and you may want to include these too. This review includes looking back and looking forward. Looking forward will lead to you setting goals and action plans for the future as part of step 3.

As part of the review on the past you could use the following questions as a framework:

- What have I done so far?
- What areas of my practice and career am I particularly proud of because I know I succeeded or overcame difficulties?

- What areas of my practice or my career am I disappointed about?
- What actions have I taken in the past to improve my practice or career and do any of these actions need to continue into the future?
- What activities have I got involved with outside work that help me develop skills I can apply to my practice or career?

There are several techniques or exercises that you can use to help you review your experience to date. An exercise that is commonly found in the profile literature is the lifeline exercise (Critten, 1996).

Lifeline exercise

This is a technique for going back through your life or career and mapping the path it has taken. It is usual to represent it as high points and low points along a time continuum. When you have drawn your line you need to mark the significant high and low points with words that indicate what was happening in your life at that time. You may find it difficult to separate personal and work-related highs and lows, and this is understandable. Although drawing the line along a time frame can be quite a superficial act, this exercise can be surprisingly powerful, especially if the highs and lows were associated with emotional times. Completing the exercise can recall those emotions and you need to be prepared for this. Making sure you have a trusted friend or colleague you can talk it through with afterwards may be helpful.

Once you have drawn the lifeline on the chart and written in the key points, look at it again. Ask yourself several questions.

- Are there sections of your career that can be put together into chunks of time because they represent particular phases in your life? How you define those phases is up to you – it could be by job titles or geographical location or by using prompts from your personal life.
- Does the lifeline tell you anything about how/why you choose to change jobs?
- Can you see any themes or pattern emerging from your life so far?

It is as important to spend time reflecting on what your lifeline shows you and writing about that as it is to do the exercise. Your reflections can begin to feed in to what you know you want to change or develop in yourself and the later stages of the profiling process.

The process of reviewing your experience to date will give you an overall picture of where you have been in the recent past and may give clues about where you need to go in the future. It may take you two or three sessions of time to do this review: the time involved depends on how much there is to say and how fast you work at thinking about it and writing it down. It needs to take as long as it needs. After the first time you complete the review you need to decide how often you do it. If where you work has an individual performance review system then you could use the review work you do for that for your UKCC profile. It is probably easiest to do a review every 6 months or when there is a change in your circumstances, e.g. leaving one job to move to another. As a minimum you should do it once a year because it will make it easier to collect them together every time you reregister.

Step 2: Self-appraisal

It always seems easier to criticize ourselves than identify what we are good at. It is important to try and develop a balanced view of self-appraisal. We're all good at some things and we all have areas that we could improve on. Self-appraisal is all about identifying both sides of this 'positive-improvement' equation. The review in step 1 should have given you broad areas of information about your career and practice. Step 2 begins to look at everything in more detail. The following questions might help.

- What do I feel is good about my self/practice?
- What do I consistently do well?
- What do I know I could improve on?
- What opportunities can I take to change my practice?
- What opportunities can I take to develop?
- What barriers will prevent me taking the opportunities?
- How can I overcome them?
- How might I sabotage myself from achieving what I want to achieve?

From time to time it will also help to reflect on particular events. These events are sometimes called critical incidents. Do not be misled by the word 'critical'. Critical incidents can be out-of-the-ordinary, life-threatening events, but they can also include day-to-day activities that are routine. Reflection and reflective practice are becoming more widespread, but there are still a lot of practitioners who feel unsure about what is meant by reflection. There are some useful references at the end of this section that will help you (Palmer *et al.*, 1994). For the purposes of building your UKCC profile they offer the following straightforward approach.

- Describe what happened, noting: any challenges which emerged; what your role was; how you felt at the time; how you dealt with the situation; and what the outcome was.
- Identify what you learnt from the situation, and reflect on how it has affected your professional development and practice.
- Consider any areas you want to develop that were highlighted by the incident.

People often get stuck writing about such incidents, because they think their writing style is poor. Remember, no one is going to mark these entries in your profile with a red pen, they are for your use only. Your style of writing or use of grammar is not the important thing here. The important thing is that writing helps you recall all the aspects of the incident more accurately and that in turn will help identify any development needs the incident raises for you.

Step 3: Setting goals and action plans

Steps 1 and 2 will have generated areas for change, improvement and development. This final step expects you to identify as specifically as possible what you are going to do about it, by when. There should be links between what you decide your learning needs are and what you choose to do with your 5 days of updating activity.

Profile maintenance and gardening!

From time to time it is important to do some weeding and tidying up and to put on the bonfire things we do not need to keep in our profile any more. You may remember that the preferred definitions of profile and portfolio both contained the word 'evidence'. You will also have gathered that profiling is about learning about yourself and from your experience.

'Evidence' and 'learning' are the two key words where profiling is concerned. There is no point in writing about a learning experience if you cannot provide evidence to support it. Conversely, there is no point including evidence of attending a study day or a practice activity if you can't show how you learnt from it and applied that learning to your practice.

Recognizing experience and converting it to evidence

Evidence is at the heart of a profile. However significant an experience might seem to you, unless you can present it in such a way that it can be verified you will not be able to get it recognized in the way you want. Do not waste time collecting material that cannot be corroborated.

For example: Write down something you have achieved in the last 6 weeks or so of which you are particularly proud. Do you have evidence of this achievement and what you learnt from it? What form does the evidence take?

The chances are that, even though you are able to find an example, finding evidence is more difficult. For example, you are asked by your manager to become involved with interviewing for new staff. Possible evidence might include:

- details of people short-listed;
- criteria the candidate had to meet to be successful;
- questions you prepared to ask at interview;
- response of interviewees;
- written summary of the discussion about which applicants to accept, dated and signed;
- any feedback about your performance;
- a commentary about how you felt about the things you did and an analysis of what you learnt from it and any future actions related to the learning.

From evidence to learning

Your evidence is only as good as the demonstration of what you have learned from it. The final stage once you have pulled all the evidence together is to look at it objectively and decide:

- what I have learnt?
- what I intend to do differently next time?
- how does it impact on my improvement action plan?

The idea of evidence equally applies to formal learning activities you might attend as part of your 5 days updating. It is not enough just to put a certificate of attendance in your profile. You need to accompany that with your reasons for attending the event – what did you hope to achieve? Where did it fit with your action plan? Then you need to document how you applied what you learnt on the day to your practice. All this information can be filed away together, along with handouts or notes you took on the day.

THE USE OF PROFILES AS PART OF THE SELECTION AND INTERVIEW PROCESS

It is becoming increasingly common for potential employers to ask those attending for interview to bring their profile with them. This is an interesting idea if managed properly, but unfortunately the implications of the idea have not always been thoroughly explored. This leads to the interviewee putting in a great deal of time and effort before the interview but the interview process not allowing time for the profile to be examined or assessed properly. If using profiles as part of the selection process is to become an increasing trend employers need to ask themselves the following questions.

- What are they trying to achieve by asking the candidates to bring their profile with them to the interview?
- Does the interview panel, or someone representing it, have the necessary knowledge and skills to assess the candidates' profiles?
- How can the panel ensure that the assessment focuses on the candidate's ability to do the job and not their skill in compiling a profile?
- How could a normally tight timescale for interviewing be increased to incorporate an effective assessment of the profile?

There is a place for using profiles as part of a selection process, particularly if the candidates do not have the exact requirements either in qualifications or experience. In this instance it is possible for the candidate to show through their profile that they have the equivalent to what would be normally expected. The emphasis could also be on transferable skills and experiences, with profile evidence showing that the candidate used skills in one situation that could also be applied to the new situation. Profiles can be used in a similar way to gain access to higher education courses by gaining credit for prior learning when the normal entrance qualifications have not been acquired.

Standard approaches taken in assessing profiles for academic purposes can also be applied to assessing them for employment purposes. The profile needs to contain evidence that the previous experience is relevant to the post being applied for, and that there is a match between the essential and desirable characteristics outlined in the job description. Hull (1997) reminds us that for academic purposes the evidence needs to have relevance, breadth, currency and authenticity; and the onus is usually placed on the candidate to present the profile material in such a way as to demonstrate these. These factors equally apply to evidence being put forward within the selection process. The evidence then needs to be assessed by someone who understands the requirements of the post being applied for and who is familiar with how to assess evidence presented within a profile.

The approach described above is a far cry from the candidate being asked to turn up with every aspect of their profile, probably more accurately called a portfolio, and the interview panel casually looking through it during the interview. The use of profiles as part of recruitment and selection can be valuable and it certainly has the potential to turn the activity away from a panel-centred process and into a candidate-centred one.

HOW CAN PROFILES BE POWERFUL?

In bringing this chapter to a close it is important to explain its title – the power of the personal professional profile. I believe that, over a period of time, the use of a profile can build the individual self-esteem of the person who owns it and, if all nurses are participating in a profiling process, the collective self-esteem of nursing as a profession.

Over a period of time, a well-kept profile provides us with a detailed map of our professional life. If we stop from time to time and review that detailed map it will show us what we have achieved professionally, how we have developed and the impact that our practice has had on us and our patients/clients. In the 'busyness' of our everyday lives we often forget what we have achieved as nurses. Instead we concentrate on what we haven't done as well as we would have liked or things that have gone completely wrong. In some perverse way, nurses always remember the worst possible times rather than the best possible times. Taking time to look at our profile redresses the balance and can remind us what a rich, successful experience we have had in our chosen profession. That reminder can be a powerful motivator, creating enthusiasm and innovation in our personal and professional lives.

REFERENCES

Boud, D., Keogh, R. and Walker, D. (1985) *Reflection: Turning Experience into Learning*, Kogan Page, London.

Brown, R. A. (1992) *Portfolio Development and Profiling for Nurses*, Quay Publishing Limited, Lancaster.

Critten, P. (1996) *Developing your Professional Portfolio*, Churchill Livingstone, Edinburgh.

Hull, C. (1997) How to get credit for previous learning. *Nursing Times*, **1** (9).

Hull, C. and Redfern, L. (1996) *Profiles and Portfolios: A Guide for Nurses and Midwives*, Macmillan, Basingstoke.

Kolb, D. (1984) *Experiential Learning: Experience as a Source of Learning and Development*, Prentice-Hall, Englewood Cliffs, NJ.

Palmer, A. M., Burns, S. and Bulman, C. (1994) *Reflective Practice in Nursing*, Blackwell Scientific, Oxford.

Redfern, L. (1997) Making a start on compiling your professional profile, learning curve. *Nursing Times*, **1**(5).

Redman, W. (1994) *Portfolios for Development: A Guide for Trainers and Managers*, Kogan Page, London.

Sheckley, B. and Keeton, M. (1994) Learning from experience. Unpublished paper given at the 1994 International Experiential Learning Conference, Washington, DC.

UKCC (1995) *UKCC's Standards for Post-registration Education and Practice (PREP), Fact Sheets 1–8*, United Kingdom Central Council for Nursing, Midwifery and Health Visiting, London.

<table>
<tr><td>

10

</td><td>

Open learning and professional development

</td></tr>
</table>

Cathy Hull

INTRODUCTION

> Today's nurses, more than at any other time, are faced with an increasing obligation to evaluate and improve their practice. The motivation to improve an individual's nursing practice may arise as an internal crusade, or it may emanate from external sources such as their peer group, their professional body or it could be politically driven. However, one thing remains clear – it is affecting, and no doubt should affect, each and every registered nurse, midwife and health visitor, regardless of where they practise and how long they have practised. (Palmer, Burns and Bulman, 1994)

Professional development involves four inter-related stages. Firstly, there is the process of coming to understand the skills, qualities and knowledge you already possess and how these can be transferred from one situation to another. The second stage involves the identification of current and future professional development goals. The third stage involves the achievement of these goals. And the final stage refers to the impact of professional development on personal practice and the environment in which practice happens. Although most professional development programmes have traditionally included at least one of these components, it is only in recent years that we have begun to see the value in including all of them. More particularly, it is the belief of those involved with the development of Macmillan Open Learning programmes that the boundaries between each of these stages are blurred, and very often the learner will be actively involved in each stage at the same time. So, for example, it is perfectly possible to reflect on past learning, identify skills, learn new skills and change professional practice at the same time.

There are several terms which can be used to refer to this process – experiential learning; flexible education; lifelong learning – Macmillan Open Learning has chosen to use the term 'open learning' as we believe this is the clearest description of the process involved.

In this chapter I shall be exploring the ways in which open learning can enhance professional development. I will be doing this from a range of perspectives, including the learning process; the management and implementation of open learning; developing an open learning curriculum and staff development issues. The aim is to encourage you to develop open approaches to professional development within your own organization, and to enable you to think through ideas about how this might be achieved.

In order to understand more about open learning, it is necessary for me to begin by introducing you to Macmillan Open Learning and giving you an idea of the context in which we are working.

MACMILLAN OPEN LEARNING – MISSION STATEMENT

Our programmes are based on the belief that the development of professional practice can only be achieved through the development of the professional as a person. We believe that:

- to become autonomous practitioners, professionals need to be self-directed autonomous learners;
- a programme of learning should focus on the learning process rather than the factual content;
- the key to learning how to learn is through enquiry, reflection, evaluation and action;
- the learner should have ownership of the learning, assessment and reflection processes;
- our programmes emphasize the integration of theory and practice in order that learners learn to structure concepts when thinking and making professional judgements in their practice;
- assessment is an integral part of the learning process, rather than separate from it, and MOL programmes:
  - enable and encourage learners to evaluate their own performance;
  - focus on learners' critical analysis skills, and their ability to apply what has been learnt;
  - enable and encourage learners to value personal theories and opinions.

ABOUT MACMILLAN OPEN LEARNING

Macmillan Open Learning (MOL) is a division of Macmillan Magazines Ltd, which publishes a range of prestigious health-care and science journals such as *Nature*, the *Health Services Journal* and the *Nursing Times*.

In 1992 MOL, in partnership with the University of Greenwich, established a professional development pathway for health-care professionals who wish to continue their personal and professional development while gaining a relevant academic award. These programmes are provided through the use of high-quality open learning materials, which are sometimes published initially through one of the Macmillan journals.

Our pathway is popular and successful and has been supported by all the relevant professional and statutory bodies. So far over 14 000 students have been registered and over 8000 have now completed. The dropout rate has been less than 2% – and reasons for doing so have largely been personal – and the pass rate is around 98%.

Our approach to learning

Our programmes are developed in the belief that education is not an incidental addition of new skills and knowledge. It is an experience that permeates all aspects of the learner's life: philosophical, cognitive, practical, emotional and social.

The philosophical components of our programmes relate to the nature of health-care professional practice – particularly nursing – and the needs of the individual learner. A primary component is a process-driven curriculum. This identifies principles and parameters by which each learner understands the steps to achieve learning outcomes. The second component is the delivery through open learning.

We believe that a process-driven curriculum delivered by an open learning system that incorporates **networking**, **facilitation** and **supervision** will meet the needs of learners who must actively reflect upon their past and current professional practice.

DIMENSIONS

There are three dimensions that underpin all of our programmes.

Practice

This involves enabling learners to reflect upon the nature of their professional practice and how standards of care can be improved. We value reflective practice, which supports learners in actively considering the day-to-day care they offer and addressing more sensitively the needs of the client or patient.

Our programmes, therefore, develop the concept of the relationship between theory and practice – which we believe to be inseparable in the delivery of care.

Person

We believe that becoming a reflective professional involves a radical and constructive review of self, which is critical for successful role change and development. The learner is therefore enabled to understand the context of her learning in response to statutory and professional changes and to explore her own motivation and values about her profession. This exploration we believe is central to the success of all professional development programmes.

Process

People learn best when they can share their ideas and develop knowledge with others. We believe that people should be encouraged to understand and use the process of group learning. By understanding their changing role as a member of student group, our learners will be equipped to negotiate the patient's care needs, employing the interpersonal and reflective skills developed in the process.

Beliefs and learning

Our materials address beliefs not only about health-care practice and the nature of role change, but also about what learners should be assisted to become. This includes:

- being capable of sustained personal and professional growth in order to develop practice wisdom (wisdom is taken to mean the distillation of knowledge and experience);
- developing as an analytical, critical reflective practitioner. We believe this is important to all professional care and to this end the integration of theory and practice and the review of experiences as a prompt to learning and change are the key concerns within our material.

Our learners are encouraged to extend the principle of reflective practice to accommodate a broader theme of informed consumerism. This entails learners actively questioning and discussing what they learn and then using this confidence to advocate the patient's rights to high-quality care or the consumer's rights to constructive health education.

The promotion of quality assurance starts with individuals insisting upon the best professional preparation for themselves, and then the best care for their clients – having learned about how 'best' may be defined.

The flexible open learning approach in our materials recognizes the learner's own commitments and empowers him/her to negotiate an individual study plan supported by a tutor/counsellor.

Facilitating and learning strategies

Our programmes allow students to develop their own programme of study depending upon their own learning needs and area of practice. The teaching and learning strategies are grounded in theories of adult learning and in particular approaches associated with open and practice-based learning. Up to 70% of study is implemented through practice.

Open learning strategies respect the rights of the learner to independence in learning, to be able to determine his/her own needs and choose the pace, time and place of his/her learning and, to some extent, the breadth and depth of the content.

This independence in learning may initially provoke anxiety in learners, especially those whose learning experience has been the traditional didactic, subject-centred, tutor-dependent approach.

Our materials do not aim to provide the definitive work on any topic. They are intended to stimulate reflection and encourage the learner to integrate his/her existing knowledge and experience with his/her developing knowledge and skills and integrate these with his/her practice.

Group work

Open learning focuses on individual learners, but we also encourage group work. Group work provides the opportunity for discussion to develop skills in both leading and working within a team.

Individual tutorials

Individual tutorials provide opportunities for the student to identify problems related to the programme and to make decisions about how best to overcome them.

Workshops

Learners attend a 2-day residential workshop each year. This helps them to network with others outside their work environment and to share knowledge and skills with others in a wider group.

Profiling

The development of a personal profile is a fundamental component of all our programmes. This is because we believe that the profiling process enables learners to develop the skills and knowledge to manage their own learning. A personal profile is simply a record of personal experience and learning that reflects the learner's development throughout the programme. The profile is used as a basis for assessing learning needs and developing a learning contract. Through profiling our learners become more aware of:

- their **attitudes and beliefs** about their chosen profession, how these have been developed and how they affect their practice;
- **life-skills**: how these have been acquired and refined and how they relate to professional practice;
- **professional strengths**, including practice skills and the knowledge and understanding that underpin them;
- **areas that need developing** to meet personal and professional needs.

This, then, is the philosophy underpinning MOL programmes. I wish now to explore this philosophy in more depth by showing how it works in practice – and in particular, through the development of our BSc (Hons) Professional Practice in Health Care.

BSC (HONOURS) PROFESSIONAL PRACTICE IN HEALTH CARE: BACKGROUND INFORMATION

In November 1995 we validated our BSc (Hons) Professional Practice in Health Care. This programme specifically recognizes the need to develop a multiprofessional approach to health-care practice. It is open to professionals who are involved in the delivery of health care, including nurses, midwives, members of the professions allied to medicine and other practitioners, for example, chiropodists and osteopaths.

Our aim was to develop a programme which would enable professionals to:

practise confidently while showing a readiness to experiment, to challenge existing practices and to take critically unconventional perspectives. In doing this they will be able to look within and beyond the context of their profession in their search for a new approach. They will seek evidence and argument through which they can justify their alternative approach thus demonstrating a scholarly approach to their practice. (University of Greenwich/Macmillan Open Learning, 1995)

So the objective is that the learner should be able to use skills of analysis, synthesis and evaluation in the way they use and develop knowledge to inform practice. These skills would also enable them to suggest creative applications for a range of concepts, which leads to them developing and extending their professional knowledge and practice.

Degree structure

This is a unitized degree programme, including core and optional units. As it is practice-based all the units are studied in conjunction with learners' experience of their field of practice. The learners' needs, therefore, and their place of work generate opportunities for the assessment of each unit and the piece of independent enquiry that forms the largest part of their assessment.

Our experience with professionals has shown that they benefit most from being able to use the pathway to enquire into their practice to solve a practice-related problem. They can do this through any of the units.

The majority registering for this award have already gained substantial degree-level credits based on their professional qualifications. These learners, therefore, need to study a further core unit, together with four option units in order to qualify for the award.

The units

Students study core and option units, which are validated at CATS level 3 as follows.

- Core unit (40 credits): Enquiring into health-care practice
- Option units (20 credits):
  - Health-care evaluation
  - Health promotion in professional practice
  - Influence in health care: media perspectives
  - Complementary therapies and health-care practice
  - Health care and the information age
  - Values and the person: ideas that influence health care
  - Professional relationships: influences on health care.

Each of these is also available to buy off the shelf in five or six separate units. This means that the student can combine topics from across the entire programme to inform and develop his/her studies. An analysis of the materials and the development process is provided later in this chapter.

Admission criteria

Our philosophy acknowledges the right of all individuals to access professional education. Nevertheless, because the programme is practice-focused it is important that the learner has access to and experience of practice. Our admission requirements, therefore, are simply that the learner should:

- hold a qualification in the health-care field that is recognized by the relevant statutory, professional or self-regulating body;
- be engaged in a relevant area of professional practice in a way that will enable him/her to meet the outcomes of the unit.

Tutor support

Students are offered comprehensive tutor support, including individual face-to-face tutorials, group tutorials, telephone support and 1-day or residential workshops. Each student has a personal tutor who supports them through the entire programme. Additional individual tutorial support is built into the programme for help with profiling, developing a learning contract and making an APEL claim. There is also an additional 12 hours tutorial support for the core unit.

The above should have given you a broad understanding of the degree programme – but how does it work in practice? Let us now move on to look at delivery of MOL programmes.

THE DELIVERY OF MOL PROGRAMMES

There are currently over 14 000 MOL registered students across the UK from as far afield as the Isle of Skye and Guernsey. Each student is linked to one of our 32 Approved Centres through a tutor/counsellor and pathway leader. The process for becoming an Approved Centre is complex and supports our quality assurance strategy.

MOL Approved Centres

Open learning needs high-quality student support and management if it is to work to the best advantage of the student. The management and delivery of our programmes, therefore, are vital to their success. With this in mind, we developed a structure in collaboration with the University of Greenwich that encourages universities, institutes of higher education and institutes of further education to seek to become an Approved Centre for our programmes. Institutions seeking approval must satisfy us that their education structure and process and assessment strategy are consistent with the quality assurance standards of the scheme.

We view the approval of a centre to offer validated materials as a partnership between MOL and the validating institution. Those involved share a common objective of providing cost-effective quality education through an open, text-based educational approach.

To ensure that this common objective is fulfilled the centre is required to follow certain procedures for approval. The organization must be:

- an organization with an academic infrastructure, which includes:
  - established educational quality assurance systems;
  - appropriate committee structures;
  - clear lines of accountability;
  - institutional quality culture;
  - corporate, rather than individual responsibility;
  - appropriate registry, student, staff, financial management information systems; and
- an organization already approved by one or more relevant professional academic validating bodies, e.g. the National Boards for nursing; the Chartered Society of Physiotherapists.

The criteria for becoming an approved centre are as follows.

- Everyone who will be involved with the programme must demonstrate a thorough understanding of the philosophy and delivery of open learning and show evidence of the implementation of this.
- Centres must demonstrate an understanding of the implications of open learning for the culture of the organization.
- Centres must articulate how providing each pathway programme supported fits into the strategic planning, including the local market, which will include individual customers as well as educational purchasers, e.g. NHS trusts.
- Centres must demonstrate how the quality assurance mechanisms are appropriate to each programme supported. This will include an appreciation of the need to resolve the tension between openness and the application of quality standards. The balance within this tension should provide academic rigour without rigidity.
- Centres are required to provide the right number of suitably qualified and experienced people who can fulfil all the roles required to run each programme and support the student during his/her programme of study, in line with the student entitlement model being used. This will include access to the appropriate subject and practice-related specialists – if applicable.
- Centres must show that students will have access to someone who has experience in supervising independent pieces of enquiry.

The centre is required to address these issues and present us with lengthy documentation for the Approvals team to digest. Once this documentation has been received an approval visit is carried out. This means that staff from MOL and the University of Greenwich (this applies only to the University of Greenwich/ Macmillan Open Learning Scheme) spend a day at the institution involved and meet:

- senior staff
- pathway leader for the programme
- tutor/counsellors
- students' managers
- students
- librarian
- external examiner
- core unit leader
- subject specialists.

The purpose of the visit is to ensure that the criteria for approval are met by the centre.

The visiting team then reports back to a Central Approvals Sub-Committee meeting where a decision regarding approval for a period of 1 or 3 years is made.

Centre support structures and staffing

Each approved centre has a management team led by the pathway leader. The management team includes representatives of all those who are involved with the programme, including tutors, students, library and computer staff.

The pathway leader is responsible for managing and implementing the programme. S/he has overall centre responsibility for the management for all MOL programmes offered within the approved centre. The workload is large and includes:

- monitoring and maintaining standards;
- recruitment of students;
- recruitment of tutors;
- staff development and initial preparation of tutors and others;
- student welfare and allocation of academic and tutor/counsellor support;
- making arrangements for the Centre Assessment Board;
- liaising with the Board of Examiners;
- monitoring and ensuring that the standard of student support is maintained by tutor/counsellors as identified in their role descriptions;
- providing annual pathway monitoring reports.

Each of these activities feeds into and informs the quality assurance mechanisms for the MOL/University of Greenwich partnership arrangements.

The process for admitting students

Once a centre has been approved, students are able to access the programme. The process through which students become registered is simple. The majority of potential students contact the Macmillan Open Learning office to request information. Once this has been sent, and the person wishes to register on the programme, MOL office staff put him/her in touch with the pathway leader based in the Approved Centre nearest to where s/he lives. The pathway leader then puts him/her in touch with a tutor/counsellor and registers him/her on the programme.

STAFF DEVELOPMENT

The skills of facilitation

Facilitating open learning requires a range of complex skills. We have identified seven core activities that facilitators use to support individuals in their personal and professional development:

- informing
- advising
- counselling

- assessing
- enabling
- advocating
- feeding back.

In practice many of these activities overlap. However, we believe that it is important to recognize the differences between them, and how one activity might be emphasized over another depending on the learning activity involved.

Often tutors who are new to open learning – and even those who have been facilitating it for some time – find it difficult to ensure that each of these activities is facilitated through an open process. At times it is much easier to revert to traditional approaches to teaching, and tell people what they should know.

Staff development workshops

We understand and sympathize with the dilemmas of facilitating an open curriculum and therefore make attending workshops a compulsory condition of becoming a tutor/counsellor. Freed from the workplace, tutor/counsellors find it valuable to share their concerns with others and debate issues to do with self-assessment, evaluation, practice-based learning, and so on.

All our new tutors attend four workshops over a 2-year period. Once they have become established MOL tutor/counsellors they attend one updating workshop per year. The first workshop is critical, because it enables the facilitator to make a final decision as to whether or not she wishes to become a tutor/counsellor. At the first workshop we:

- introduce the philosophy of open learning;
- begin to identify skills in distance teaching – such as telephone tuition and feedback;
- familiarize tutor/counsellors with the degree programme;
- familiarize the tutor/counsellor with the resources available;
- establish support groups.

Three more workshops are run at intervals throughout a 2-year period, which enables the tutor/counsellor to continue the learning process by evaluating his/her role and identifying and solving problems.

We also encourage Approved Centres to offer their own professional development programme, and many of our centres have done this. One centre, for example, holds twice-yearly 'awaydays' where our tutor/counsellors and others involved with open learning programmes across the organization come together to share ideas and debate issues.

THE CURRICULUM FRAMEWORK

Another unique element of delivery is that the materials that support the programme are not compulsory reading. Rather, we encourage our learners to use all the facilities of the institution in which they are based and beyond, to read widely and not to follow the materials in a dogged or rigid fashion. Our materials are generic, and written in the knowledge that each student will be supported by a tutor – who will help them to make their learning relevant to their individual needs and encourage them to read beyond the text presented.

The materials, then, emphasize profiling, learning contracts and the acquisition of study skills appropriate to the needs of adult learners.

Let us now move on to look at the development of the curriculum framework in more depth.

Developing the curriculum framework

The rationale

The rationale behind the development of our BSc (Hons) Professional Practice in Health Care was the awareness that health-care professionals now need to keep up to date and continue their professional education throughout their career. Health services are rapidly changing and place increasing demands on professional staff. Staff are now expected to be innovative, flexible, resourceful, adaptable, self-reliant and responsible for their actions. All these expectations can only be achieved if health-care professionals are encouraged to continue their education in a way that encourages them to apply their learning directly to their field of practice.

Degree-level professional development

Because we were developing a professional development qualification, the degree team felt it was important to agree on a definition of degree level 3 work that would support professional work and inform the design of the curriculum framework. We came up with the following:

> (Level 3) Practitioners are specialists within their chosen areas, who have developed new professional skills, knowledge and understanding; who have utilized existing research; whose practice is enquiry based and who promote innovative practice. (University of Greenwich/Macmillan Open Learning, 1995)

Within this definition is the recognition that our learners are encouraged to apply and reflect on the content of the learning materials in relation to their own area of practice. Our programmes are based on the belief that professionals learn best when they are self-directed and their learning is related to and arises from their experience and current practice.

So our programmes are based on a process-driven curriculum – students choose what they want to learn, how they want to learn and where they want to learn it. Developing the materials that promote a process-driven curriculum of this type is complex and requires enormous expertise, including subject specialists, academic and professional staff, text-based designers and others. There were over 70 people involved in the design and development of each stage of the BSc (Hons) Professional Practice in Health Care, and the following teams were established:

- **the core team**, with overall responsibility for the development of the degree programme, from idea to finished product;
- **the degree team** responsible for developing the degree framework;
- **subject specialist teams** responsible for the development of individual units;
- **critical readers** with responsibility for the entire degree programme;
- **critical readers** responsible for individual units;
- **development testers** responsible for individual units;
- **the design team**.

The materials development process itself is complex, and a diagrammatic representation of it is shown in Figure 10.1.

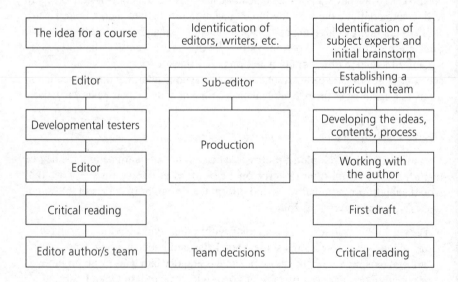

Figure 10.1 Materials development process

THE MATERIALS

In designing the support material we began by acknowledging that each of us learns in different ways – we therefore needed to develop material that would support the needs of individual learners; as one of my colleagues put it: 'we offer 1000 programmes for 1000 different learners' (Marianne Phillips, Head of Division, Macmillan Open Learning).

The team thought carefully about what motivates people to learn and how they learn best – particularly if they are busy professionals with little time to spare. We thought about what creates effective teaching and learning, and we came up with a list that looked something like this.

- There may be a charismatic tutor.
- People are in control.
- Students determine their own needs.
- Students are learning from each other.
- Students feel motivated to read more.
- The material presented is relevant and up to date.
- The material draws upon personal as well as professional experience.
- Learning should not be held back by discipline boundaries.
- Creativity; action; energy.

The problem for the team was how to incorporate all of these ideas within the pages of a book. We decided that the layout of the material was as important as style, language and content. And our solution was to think carefully about what the page itself would look like.

Each book is divided into five or six sections, with each section divided into topics. Most topics take up two facing pages – a double page spread. Learners are to read the book in this way – looking at both pages together as a whole. On each page there are large spaces – this is to encourage the learner to make notes and brainstorm ideas. It also reminds the reader that the book is a dynamic tool for learning – it does not contain precious words that need to be kept safe. Rather, it provides some ideas to motivate and excite the learner.

The top half of the page contains the kind of information that will stimulate the learner into researching and finding out more about the topic. The bottom half of the page has different sorts of information and gives the learner the opportunity to do something with it. There are activities, diagrams, discussion points, quotes, references, charts, current debates, case studies and ideas for assessment topics.

However, the learner can read the bottom half of the page before the top half or mix them in a way that helps them to think and learn. It is very difficult to give you a true flavour of the materials within this chapter as the materials are designed to be seen on double A4 pages. However, the two pages of materials shown in Figure 10.2 should give you an idea of how the design works.

The materials also include things that will draw on the learner's experience and have personal meaning. So, for example, this poem has been incorporated into the appropriate behaviour change. This 'propaganda' view of information exchange was enthusiastically espoused by the Central Council for Health Education in the 1930s and '40s (see pages 18–19). As it became increasingly clear that this did not work, the metaphor changed from a syringe to an aerosol: 'as you spray it on the surface, some of it hits the target, most of it drifts away, and very little of it penetrates' (Mendelsohn, 1968).

The pendulum has now swung back to somewhere between these two models: use of the mass media can be a powerful ally or a weak partner. It depends on the 'fit' between message and medium: the strength of a message, the way it is put across, and most important of all — how receptive the audience is. What is now clear is that it is much easier to raise people's awareness of an issue than it is actually to change their behaviour in response to that issue. For example, an analysis of the response to the government's major AIDS campaign in the spring of 1987 revealed a clear rise in the following two to three months. But there was no discernible change in sexual behaviour and people who knew most about the syndrome perceived their own risk of contracting it as having reduced over the period (Wober, 1988). Similarly, alcohol education programmes launched through the media frequently produce a change in knowledge about the risks of alcohol but rarely have much influence on drinking behaviour

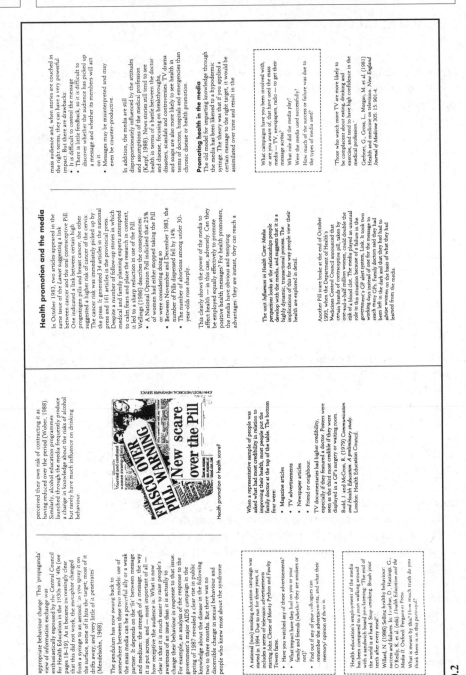

Health promotion or health scare?

A national (non) smoking education campaign was started in 1994. Due to run for three years, it includes a series of television advertisements starring John Cleese of Monty Python and Fawlty Towers fame.
- Have you watched any of these advertisements?
- What impact have they had on you or your family and friends (whether they are smokers or not)?
- Find out if any of your colleagues can remember the advertisements, and what their memory/opinion of them is.

Health education's employment of the media has been compared to a man walking around with a sandwich board proclaiming 'The end of the world is at hand. Stop smoking. Brush your teeth after every meal!'.
Willard, N. (1986) Selling healthy behaviour: success and failures. In: J. Cather, D. Hastings, G. O'Reilly, K. et al. (eds.) *Health Education and the Media II*. Oxford: Pergamon Press.
What is meant by this? How much truth do you think there is in this portrayal?

Health promotion and the media

In October 1983, two articles appeared in the same issue of the *Lancet* suggesting a link between cancer and the oral contraceptive Pill. One indicated a link between certain high progestogen pills and breast cancer, the other suggested a higher risk of cancer of the cervix. The cancer risk was immediately picked up by the press. It generated 34 articles in the national press and 161 articles in the provincial press. Despite a number of follow-up stories in which medical and family planning experts attempted to calm fears and place the research in context, it led to a sharp reduction in use of the Pill. Wellings (1986) describes how:
- A National Opinion Poll indicated that 25% of women had either stopped taking the Pill or were considering doing so
- Between November and December 1983, the number of Pills dispensed fell by 14%
- The number of abortions among under 30-year-olds rose sharply.

This clearly shows the power of the media to affect health — in this case, adversely. Can they be employed equally effectively to promote positive health messages? For health promoters, the media have obvious and tempting advantages: they are instant, they can reach a mass audience and, when stories are couched in the right terms, they can have a very powerful impact. But there are drawbacks.
- It is difficult to control the message
- There is little feedback, so it is difficult to discover whether the audience has picked up a message and whether its members will act on it
- Messages may be misinterpreted and may even be counter-productive.

In addition, the media are still disproportionately influenced by the attitudes and assumptions of the medical profession (Karpf, 1988). News stories still tend to see health in terms of a battle between the doctor and disease, focusing on breakthroughs, disasters, scandals and controversies. TV drama and soaps are also more likely to see health in terms of doctors, hospitals and emergencies than chronic disease or health promotion.

Promoting health in the media
The old model for imparting knowledge through the media has been likened to a hypodermic syringe. The theory was that if you applied a certain message to the right target, it would be assimilated over time and result in the

The unit *Influences in Health Care: Media perspectives* looks at the relationships people develop with the media, and suggests that it is a highly dynamic, transactional process. The implications of this for the way people view their health are explored in detail.

Another Pill scare broke at the end of October 1995, when the Department of Health's Medicines Control Council announced that certain brands of contraceptive pill, taken by one-and-a-half million women, could double the risk of a blood clot. The media played an initial role in this situation because of a failure in the government's GP alert system. Link. It took two working days instead of one for the message to reach many GPs. Family doctors said they had been left in the dark and that they had had to advise women on the basis of what they had learned from the media.

- What campaigns have you been involved with, or are you aware of, that have used the mass media — TV, newspapers, radio — to get their message across?
- What role did the media play?
- Were the media used successfully?
- How much of the success or failure was due to the types of media used?

Those who watch more TV are more likely to be complacent about eating, drinking and exercise, and tend to have high confidence in the medical profession.
Gerbner, G, Gross, L, Morgan, M. et al. (1981) Health and medicine on television. *New England Journal of Medicine* 305: 15: 901–4.

Figure 10.2

materials at a stage when the student is most likely to be feeling vulnerable and unsure of his/her ability to learn:

> Apollinaire said
> 'Come to the edge'
> 'But it is too high'
> 'Come to the edge'
> 'We might fall'
> 'Come to the edge'
> And they came
> And he pushed them
> And they flew. (Anonymous, in Cope, 1994)

The materials, therefore, are constructed in a way that allows people to dip in and out of them according to their needs. Some people like to start at the beginning of a book and work through to the end. Others prefer a less systematic approach and like to take in different points of view as they go along. From the outset we tell the learner that links between sections are built into the text, and they may find themselves going from one section to another. There is no particular reason to read the various sections in the order in which they are presented.

REFLECTIVE PRACTICE

The materials encourage learners to reflect on the new ideas coming into their minds and how the specific and generic knowledge they acquire can be related to practice. We believe that 'reflection is a generic term for learning' (Boud, Keogh and Walker, 1985) and there are no right or wrong ways as to how reflection might occur. Learners, therefore, might reflect by having a conversation with themselves or with other people.

> But it is a particular sort of conversation: asking questions, explaining, disagreeing, trying to get to the heart of the matter, turning things over in your mind, worrying about them. (MOL, 1997)

We also emphasize the importance of writing as a tool for learning. Students write some of their conversations down in a learning journal or reflective diary. They might be writing about:

- the process of learning;
- the consequences of what has been learned;
- what they have discovered about themselves as they learn.

We encourage learners to feed uncertainties into their writing and discussions and to use their personal profile as a means for doing this.

Profiling

The assessment process is integral to the design and delivery of all of our programmes. Assessment in the widest sense enables learners to keep track of their professional development – and to work out what they are learning and how this can be used. One way of undergoing self-assessment is through keeping a personal professional profile. Profiling can provide a rich resource for reflecting upon what has been learned, which can be drawn upon at a later date, such as when planning and producing written assessments.

Profiling draws upon experience and encompasses many different styles of writing. Profiling includes informal writing – the sort that is written in a learning journal or log – which offers the learner the chance to be creative and imaginative without worrying about presenting ideas for others to read and/or assess.

It is our belief that writing, reflection and learning feed into one another and cannot be easily separated. So, in the introduction to the materials we say:

> As you examine your work, writing down your thoughts will help you to make connections between learning, feeling and doing. This kind of informal writing helps you discover what you think about complex topics and will help you to write better formal assessments. (MOL, 1997)

Profiling, then, helps the learner and others to make sense of what they are learning and to relate this to their personal and professional life. It is a structured process of reflecting upon skills and knowledge and planning current and future career and professional development needs. Profiling helps learners to analyse their experience and view this more critically. It also helps them to appreciate their own professional development and value the breadth and depth of their existing knowledge.

> Profiling means keeping a record of these things, organized in a way that is clear to you. Most profiles include a fair bit of writing, because this is a good way of keeping a record and because writing things down often helps to clarify them in your mind. Writing can also help you make connections between different aspects of your life and learning. (MOL, 1997)

Macmillan Open Learning publishes a Profile Pack, which students on the degree programme are able to buy, although it is not compulsory to do so. At the time of going to print this remains the most popular profile pack on the market and is used by a range of people working in a variety of contexts. It provides a structure for learners to understand and appreciate the significance of what and how they learn, enhances their self-awareness and builds confidence. It also offers them an effective and up-to-date record of their past and current learning, and provides a powerful means of communication with employers, present and future (MOL, 1993).

ASSESSMENT

It is an essential element of all MOL programmes that the learner is actively involved in the assessment process. The learner should be encouraged to think critically about what s/he is learning, to identify standards and criteria that apply to his/her professional practice, and to evaluate the extent to which these criteria have been met. There is a commitment that all assessment will have a formative, developmental component. The materials encourage the learner to think about assessment as soon as possible: 'You take charge of assessment – within the limits of the BSc programme and what you agree with your tutor/counsellor after negotiation' (MOL, 1997).

As the degree is practice-based and all the units are studied in conjunction with the learners' experience of their field of practice, it is the needs of the learner and his/her place of work that generate opportunities for the assessment of each unit. Our experience with professional development has shown that learners benefit most when the learning is made relevant to their individual needs. So, there may be work-based imperatives that drive them towards using the opportunity to enquire into their practice to solve a practice-related problem.

Learning outcomes

Students undertaking the degree need to show that they can:

* critically reflect on and challenge existing practice;
* draw on perspectives from within and beyond their own chosen professional boundaries and use these to inform their own practice, where appropriate;
* develop and extend their own professional knowledge and skills through a process of analysis, synthesis and evaluation of the contemporary theoretical concepts that underpin practice;
* plan, conduct and evaluate an enquiry-based project related to their field of practice;
* critically reflect on and evaluate their own personal, professional development and learning.

These are the overall learning outcomes for the degree programme as a whole. However, each unit has specific learning outcomes attached. So, for example, for the unit Health-care Evaluation, specific learning outcomes include the following.

* Discuss the origins and development of health-care evaluation from a variety of perspectives.
* Critically review a range of concepts and models of health-care evaluation.
* Evaluate your own personal and professional practice in relation to health-care evaluation.

A learning contract

In order to help students to achieve these learning outcomes, they develop a learning contract, which is shared with their tutor counsellor.

We believe that there is no right or wrong way of writing a learning contract. People learn and write in different ways. However, we do encourage people to try writing different ones before finding the one that suits them best.

The profile forms the basis from which the learner, in conjunction with his/her tutor/counsellor, develops a learning contract to guide him/her through the degree pathway. Such a contract is a dynamic tool central to the learning process and it is revised when and where necessary as the student progresses through his/her studies.

Our approach to writing a learning contract is based on the idea that it is a learning agreement between two or more people – primarily student and tutor/counsellor. The aim of the contract is simply to help learners to clarify their ideas, devise realistic objectives and keep track of changes. Students might choose not to write down their learning contract – although they usually do as it helps in clarifying and ordering your thoughts.

The work done in a personal profile will help the learner to develop a learning contract. This is because, as learners think about what they have done in the past and what they are doing now, they begin to identify what they wish to learn in the future – in both the short and long term. The learning contract should therefore include these long- and short-term goals. The learning contract shown in Figure 10.3 is based on that developed by one of our learners.

So, through profiling and the development of a learning contract learners are able to identify the areas they wish to develop for personal, professional or academic reasons.

> The areas for development form the basis of a goal-setting process in which they define the goal, set criteria by which it can be assessed and develop an action plan for achieving those criteria. This activity is central to the learning process throughout the programme and for the degree pathway it is particularly crucial in helping the student construct their own relevant and coherent programme of study. (University of Greenwich/Macmillan Open Learning, 1995)

OPEN LEARNING AND PROFESSIONAL PRACTICE

In May 1997, the new government appointed a Minister for Lifelong Learning, Kim Howells. This is because the government quickly recognized that the concept of lifelong learning is fundamental to the development of professionals and citizens alike. The ENB (1994) described lifelong learners as:

LEARNING CONTRACT

Re: Section 2
What do I need to do?

1 Use the next three weeks to work through the unit.
2 Plan time in my diary to vist the library to follow up references.
3 Attend group tutorial.
4 Make one appointment with tutor/counsellor to discuss ideas I have about my assessment.

What am I trying to learn from this Section? (to be discussed with tutor/counsellor after group tutorial)

1 *The Black Report and The Health Divide* seem to be important references in health inequalities. I need to try to understand more about the effect of poverty on health by:
   • Making notes from these books
   • Finding a copy of more recent articles on health inequalities
   • Asking Sally, Andrew and Jenny (fellow students) to take part in a discussion about health inequalities.
2 During Section 1, I found myself skipping some of the suggested Activities. It didn't seem to matter at first, but Sally says she gets more out of the material by doing them. I'll set myself a target to do 50% of them for Section 2 and then evaluate it.

LEARNING CONTRACT

This is the first time I've ever learnt this way and I keep getting lost and feeling I'm not achieving anything. A colleague suggested I make a definite plan – what I'm going to learn – and then agree it with my tutor/counsellor. I decided to try it for Sections 1 and 2.

1 Go through, page by page, and mark up any references I need to follow up.
   Action: Book time to go to the library.
2 Not sure about the difference between health education and health promotion. Is there any real difference or is it just words?
   Action: Need to explore this with colleagues.
3 Don't understand the explanation of paradigms. Need to understand it before I go on with the unit.
   Action: Follow up the references and discuss at tutorial group meeting.
4 Interested in the link between poor health and poverty.
   Action: Find out whether any initiatives exist in my area to combat health inequalities.

Figure 10.3

• innovative in their practice
• flexible to changing demand
• resourceful in their methods of working
• able to work as change agents
• able to share good practice and knowledge
• adaptable to changing health-care needs
• challenging and creative in their practice
• self-reliant in their way of working
• responsible and accountable for their actions.

It is very likely that health-care professionals will be expected to achieve these characteristics through their own learning initiative – and not simply from sitting in a classroom and being filled up with knowledge. Professional development, then, is a lifelong learning process, which involves the elements shown in Figure 10.4.

- Reflecting on your past experience – to identify skills, knowledge and qualities
- Identifying current and future personal and professional educational and career-related needs
- Learning new knowledge, changing attitudes and beliefs
- Developing a framework for achieving these learning goals

Figure 10.4 The lifelong learning process

Implicit in this approach is the notion that professional development is a continual cycle, which encourages people to change and adapt their professional practice in response to the ever-changing scene of today's health service. It also recognizes that personal and professional development needs are not always separate. In recent years, professionals have recognized that it is not easy to separate what we learn from our personal life from what we learn as professionals. Rather, our values about our professional practice are often influenced by attitudes and beliefs we hold in other aspects of our life. This is something that our learners quickly recognize as they work on their profile:

> When I began my profile I was fairly sceptical. What a lot of work for nothing, I thought. What does it matter what I think about when I am off duty, what really matters is what I do on the ward? I found doing the profile quite a challenge – although when I got further into it I was surprised by how much of what I do at home has informed my practice. I now think much more about what I believe in and hold good – and this has helped me to think about the nature of my practice and my role in it. (A student on a MOL programme)

Most of us base our understanding of ourselves upon what other people tell us and their perception of us, the so-called 'looking-glass self'. However, these perceptions might not be accurate and are therefore not sufficient on their own for the development of true self-awareness. In order to achieve this, we also need to engage in a process of introspection, i.e. to look within ourselves and attempt to recognize, and own, our feelings and reactions. By this means we may avoid developing a false sense of self.

A NOTE ABOUT CREDIT

Open learning enables people to understand more about themselves and their educational needs. It also offers a way of enabling others to recognize the learner's skills and experience.

Clearly, getting credit for all of our learning, wherever and however this has been acquired, is an important element in recognizing the value of our informal, personal knowledge. Within the MOL/University of Greenwich pathway it is possible for learners to enter the degree programme with advanced standing of up to 260 credit points. This includes advanced standing for their licence-to-practise qualification but also includes accreditation of prior learning (APL) and prior experiential learning (APEL).

The APEL system operating within the scheme is a centralized University of Greenwich system. This involves the use of distance learning materials plus personal counselling from an APEL counsellor. Examples of evidence for an APEL claim include:

- reflective writing;
- health-care plans;
- appropriate workplace assessment;
- projects or articles.

In this way, APEL draws on the individual's personal experience and integrates it with his/her professional practice.

While we acknowledge the excellence of some institution-focused professional development provision, the opportunity to attend on-campus courses as full-time or part-time students is rare for most health-care professionals. Rather, staff are now keen to undertake professional development that has relevance to the workplace and helps to solve real issues and problems. In this way what is learned is integrated into practice to the benefit of learner, patient/client and organization alike. The flexibility of open learning enables these issues to be addressed by offering health-care professionals the chance to study at graduate level through a process-driven open curriculum that builds on their experience. The flexibility of the MOL degree also means that learners have the opportunity to select units that, because they are generic, can always be related to their individual development needs. Time and again students completing our programme say: 'I didn't realize I knew so much. I didn't realize I could do so much' (Hull, 1993). For many, it is also the first time that their professional role has been recognized. At a recent reapproval visit, one student who had recently completed said:

The first person to value my nursing skills was my tutor/counsellor. She made me feel that I had a lot to offer the profession and I was capable of achieving a lot. This gave me confidence in myself – and I haven't looked back. Now I have finished the MOL diploma I intend to do the degree. Before I started the diploma I thought I was stupid.

In our approach to open learning the gap between theory and practice is narrow. This doesn't mean that nursing is the only subject studied. Rather, open learning breaks down barriers to learning, including the barriers we as learners build for ourselves that stop us from learning and developing, as well as the barriers that institutions and professions erect, which serve to contain knowledge within a very narrow definition. Through open learning, professionals are encouraged to become reflective practitioners who can think for themselves and make informed decisions. Moreover, what has always interested me about professional education is that it often appears very flat and dry. By that I mean that people do not approach it with the same level of enthusiasm that they approach other courses, hobbies and activities. What is exciting about open learning is that it is eclectic and values all learning – wherever it happens. People can and do bring their interests, values and passions to their professional development through this process.

I have seen people get really excited and passionate about doing their profiles, in the same way as I have seen them excited about reading a novel or painting a picture. For my part, what I want to hold good is that open learning offers an approach to professional development that makes people passionate about seeking knowledge, about finding out about themselves and about going out into the world and learning new things. I want nurses and midwives to experience the excitement and commitment to knowledge that makes professional learning desirable, and thereby much more human.

REFERENCES

Boud, D., Keogh, R. and Walker, D. (1985) *Reflection: Turning Experience into Learning*, Kogan Page, London.
Cope, W. (1994) *Poem for the Day*, Sinclair-Stevenson, London
Hull, C. (1993) Making experience count, in *Learner Managed Learning: Practice, Theory and Policy*, (ed. N. Graves), Higher Education for Capability, Leeds.
MOL (1993) *The Profile Pack*, Macmillan Open Learning, London.
MOL (1997) *Introductory Unit to BSc(Hons) Professional Practice in Health Care*, Macmillan Open Learning, London
Palmer, A., Burns, S. and Bulman, C. (1994) *Reflective Practice in Nursing: the Growth of the Professional Practitioner*, Blackwell, Oxford.
University of Greenwich/Macmillan Open Learning (1995) *Definitive Pathway Document for BSc (Hons) Professional Practice in Health Care*, Macmillan Open Learning, London.

The accreditation of prior learning and nurse education in higher education

11

Christine Butterworth and Linda Thorne

Processes to give professional and academic credit for health practitioners' learning at work are an accepted feature of many qualifying courses for the health professions. This chapter will look in detail at some current examples of such processes in higher education in the UK. Before looking at specific examples, however, it is helpful to look at the accreditation of prior learning (AP(E)L) in a broader context.

We have used the acronym AP(E)L to include both certificated (APL) and uncertificated experiential prior learning. This is consistent with the usage of the South East England Consortium for Credit Accumulation and Transfer (SEEC), the body producing guidelines for AP(E)L practice in higher education.

AP(E)L is an international phenomenon: it has a place in many national policies aiming to assist lifelong learning. There are broad questions that are worth asking in order to understand this phenomenon: why has its spread been so rapid? How is its implementation affected by the political and social context in which it is developed? There are also questions that practitioners will want to focus on: what are the advantages that AP(E)L seems to offer? Equally important, as information about the implementation of AP(E)L begins to be collected: what similarities and differences are there in the way it is implemented in different places?

THE PLACE OF AP(E)L IN HIGHER EDUCATION IN THE UK

For a large part of the educational history of the UK, adult education and training have been marginal activities, outside the mainstream of compulsory and higher education. Since the 1980s, this has changed. The public statements of many interested parties – government, the professions, business and industry – now place prime importance on continuing education and training for adults.

This shift is driven by national concerns about the need to remain competitive in global markets, and by forecasts that technological and economic changes will make employees' skills date faster than ever before. (One US estimate is that half the workforce's skills go out of date every 3–5 years.) Lifelong learning has become a social and economic mission of many governments, the UK included.

The same period has seen a huge expansion in the UK higher education (HE) system, with the incorporation of the polytechnics and their move to university status. Several occupations (including, of course, nursing and other health-care occupations) are now restructuring themselves and using higher education to become graduate professions, and there have been many innovations in work-based learning and continuing professional development (CPD).

These developments have been made possible by, and themselves stimulated, significant changes in the structure of the HE curriculum, producing a debate that seeks to redefine the purpose(s) of HE in the context of these changes (Barnett, 1990) and, by association, to identify the skills, knowledge and values with which its graduates are equipped (UDACE, 1991).

The major change in the structure of the higher education curriculum, at least as far as the ex-polytechnics were concerned, was the shift from year-based degree and diploma courses to accreditation frameworks with programmes delivered as units and credits, with levels of qualification formally defined.

This structural change created the possibility of giving credit for part-completion of courses, and for relevant qualifications and experiences gained before entering higher education. Before it was wound up, the validating body for these newest universities, the CNAA, published guidelines for AP(E)L schemes, influenced by practice in the USA during the 1970s (CNAA, 1988). The justification for the development of AP(E)L in the USA was the need to widen access to higher education, to support the recruitment of people without 'traditional' qualifications for entry.

The same purpose was, unsurprisingly, advocated by British commentators as AP(E)L schemes appeared in a fast-expanding higher education system. In an otherwise gloomy review of British adult and continuing education during the 'devastation' of the 1980s and early 1990s (when the government lowered student support in higher education while increasing numbers, reduced support for mature students and shifted funding from non-vocational further and adult education to vocational), Stock (1996) nevertheless noted approvingly the promise that AP(E)L offered of widening access. Barnett (1990) applauded its radical potential, and asserted that AP(E)L was an element in the enlarged definition of 'academic freedom' appropriate to the new expanded higher education – it was a student's right to have previous relevant experiential learning taken account of by higher education's gatekeepers.

This is the context in which nurse education became part of higher education during the late 1980s and 1990s – a sector experiencing considerable innovation and rapid expansion, both of its student body and of its mission towards those students. In the vocational and professional areas that employed the graduates of these universities, for whom higher education provided CPD through higher degrees and diplomas, the same period saw a series of innovations at the interface of professional experience and formal CPD. These developments aimed to update the knowledge and skills of employees, and also to widen the student base of the institutions. Before going into further detail about AP(E)L in the UK, however, it will be useful to take a brief look at some international developments during the same period.

THE DEVELOPMENT OF AP(E)L IN OTHER HIGHER EDUCATION SYSTEMS

The USA is the accepted 'home' of AP(E)L, which began with schemes to facilitate the access to higher education of troops returning from the Second World War. Its spread during the late 1970s established the general feasibility of giving higher education credit for informal or experiential learning. By the 1990s there were over 1700 colleges and universities offering AP(E)L, and a major professional organization, the Council on Adult Experiential Learning, supporting AP(E)L developments and working to extend higher education's recognition of work-based learning. The higher education system in the USA is, of course, diverse and very large. In countries with smaller systems it is noticeable that AP(E)L is seen, in the current economic context of higher education, as a potentially valuable element in the development of nationally coordinated systems of education and training.

Australia

A report commissioned by the Australian Vice-Chancellors' Committee (Cohen *et al.*, 1993) gave the findings of a survey which showed that AP(E)L (called RPL: Recognition of Prior Learning in Australia and New Zealand) was 'well-established', with virtually three-quarters of Australian universities having some kind of RPL scheme. The RPL that existed up to the time of that report was mainly offered to facilitate transfer between higher education courses and give credit for certificated learning. The report was part of the Australian government's plans to establish a national credit framework articulating the HE and FE sectors (similar to the UK government's plans for NCVQ).

The report's authors were keen to make the case that it was 'sound educational practice' to extend RPL procedures to cover experiential, uncertificated or work-based learning. They recommended three main principles on which Australian higher education should develop RPL. In common with the USA and UK justifications for such processes, they stressed the 'equity access' principle: assisting 'non-traditional' higher education entrants into higher education. They also believed that an extension of RPL would stimulate debate about their second principle: 'quality' in higher education, which can be interpreted as a belief that the extension of RPL would force a curriculum debate about the definitions of levels and standards (something that was well advanced in many UK universities by this time). Their final principle was an important instrumental one: 'efficiency', i.e. RPL accelerated students' progress through courses, thus saving them and their sponsors or employers time and money. This use of RPL/APE(E)L has become a central element in the picture of AP(E)L in the cash-strapped 1990s, as will become clear in the accounts that follow.

New Zealand

RPL in New Zealand is supported by the government as part of the national policy for training and education. The New Zealand Qualifications Authority (NZQA) was required by an education act of 1990 to include recognition of 'competency already achieved'. Like the UK's NCVQ, the NZQA framework is based on standards developed by groups from education, the professions and industry but, in contrast to NCVQ, the New Zealand framework aimed to include all sectors of education from its inception, secondary, tertiary and higher, in a 'seamless' system.

In 1993 the NZQA published national guidelines for RPL policy and practice, and university staff were prominent in a newly established group of practitioners: the RPL Institute, initiating research and development. As in Australia, various undocumented university procedures for assessing relevant previous experiences (e.g. part-completion of courses, establishing the equivalence of courses completed overseas) already existed: 'a climate conducive to RPL is part of the New Zealand university culture' (Harre Hindmarsh, 1992). From the first, RPL was seen as one current in 'the ocean of Lifelong Learning' (Hornblow, 1995) and those involved were able to take advantage of evaluative research into existing models and practices. The 'social justice' ideal of widening access was a founding principle, but writers also noted that some RPL schemes took advantage of 'niche marketing', targeting mature employees keen to fast-track their way to professional qualifications by RPL portfolios – what one researcher called the 'marketization model' (Hornblow, 1995) because of the amount of fees it generated.

France

AP(E)L development in France is, as in the previous examples, also stimulated by government policy but, unlike them, is not linked to the systematic development of national qualifications frameworks. Here too, AP(E)L is founded on the principles of social justice (i.e. widening access to higher education) and supporting employability, including movement between European universities.

Policy distinguished two concepts, recognition and accreditation, as separate, though linked, and established procedures to support the extension of a system of recognition of prior learning (which does not include certification/accreditation) as part of adult education to help individuals develop career plans and negotiate access to education, training or jobs. It is up to individuals to secure their own accreditation with institutions.

As in other countries, there was a limited historical precedent for AP(E)L: there had been a scheme for over 50 years that allowed experienced technicians advanced standing towards engineering degrees, though the numbers were very small. Driven by the same economic forces as the other education and training systems in the 1980s, the Ministry of Education decreed in 1985 that universities should set up procedures to support access by students without the traditional bac-calaureate. Universities proved resistant, and this requirement was enforced by law in 1992, enabling any individual with 5 years of work experience (not life experi-ence) to gain advanced standing towards a degree. From 1994 procedures were developed with universities, companies and education authorities. The present sit-uation is that about one-third of universities apply AP(E)L, notably those (e.g. Lille, Grenoble) with a tradition of adult education and professional training.

The French model concentrates on the process of 'recognition'. This is carried out in 120 centres (*centres de bilan*) staffed by interdisciplinary teams: educa-tion/training specialists, psychologists and human resources specialists. Some cen-tres have links with regional groups of universities. The basis of the French model is a 'competence audit' (*bilan de competence*) which is the individual's develop-ment plan, compiled as a 'dossier'. The range of methods of assessing candidates' skills and experiences are familiar ones in AP(E)L practice: interviews, self-assessment tests, portfolio. Where appropriate, assessment is done by university subject specialists.

The distinctive features of this model lie in the fact that it is carried out outside higher education (not by the gatekeepers), and in its emphasis on the career plan-ning which follows the reflection on and articulation of the individual's previous experiences, learning and achievements. The access issue is not stressed as much as in the other systems described above, perhaps because in France a bigger pro-portion of the school population leaves with qualifications fit for entry to higher education:

In France, [AP(E)L] is likely to be considered more as a route to lifelong learning than a second chance because about 70% of a certain age group achieve the baccalaureate level. (Barkatoolah, 1997)

COMMON FEATURES OF AP(E)L DEVELOPMENT

What has this brief review of international AP(E)L development established?

First, that in all higher education systems, some kind of precedent for recognizing relevant informal learning already existed. Whether formal but limited or an occasional university admissions practice, the principle was familiar. What is new is the scale: education policies now clearly acknowledge the potential value of AP(E)L as one of a range of strategies with a contribution to make to lifelong learning, and are giving it a high profile.

Secondly, however high profile the policy, the relative autonomy of higher education does not ensure a simple 'implementation' of AP(E)L schemes. Accrediting off-campus learning, whether via AP(E)L or work-based learning programmes, challenges the autonomy of higher education, and universities –and professional bodies – are often, at least initially, sceptical of AP(E)L as a development that might dilute academic standards.

Thirdly, a point that follows from the last one: AP(E)L has made a particular contribution in stimulating innovation and debate about the HE curriculum and CPD. To enable formal assessment of past learning to be matched with the learning expected from course completion, the standards and outcomes of those courses have to be articulated and visible to students as well as staff.

Fourthly, though the essential principles of AP(E)L may be shared internationally, the models that develop are affected by their national context. There is a contrast between, for example, French and UK developments. In France the AP(E)L centres were centrally initiated, partly as a reaction to universities dragging their feet: the government could compel employers to subsidize personal and career development by means of a levy but it could not compel universities to accredit the process. In the UK, by contrast, AP(E)L in HE is practitioner-led from within the higher education institutions themselves, much as curriculum development progressed in schools before the centralized National Curriculum, i.e. there is variety in schemes according to how practitioners in a particular institution interpret the needs of their clients.

AP(E)L IN UK UNIVERSITIES

Although the autonomy of HE means that it can choose what it will accredit, other educational policy created a market for HE institutions and an economic context for HE (and FE) in which they compete for students. A recent UCAS survey of AP(E)L in higher education (UCAS, 1996) indicates the part AP(E)L is able to play in this market. All institutions in the UCAS system were questioned on their use of AP(E)L, and the results confirm the trends noted in the above discussion. There is a variety of practice, based on the institutions' 'own missions, admissions policies and programme structures' (UCAS, 1996). This variety includes students being able to claim AP(E)L for access to courses or to gain academic credit through AP(E)L to get advanced standing on courses. This advanced standing may be in the form of general credit that simply shortens their time to the award or of specific credit that gives exemption from particular course modules or units.

One part of the F/HE sector has a tradition of offering courses to 'non-traditional' or 'second-chance' groups such as access students, refugees or mature returners without entry qualifications. In this sector the spread of AP(E)L is due to the fact that its processes are based on values that 'fit' with the culture of this sector of provision. These values include a commitment to supporting the personal as well as academic development of the student, and to extending access and choice to groups neglected by most of HE. This is one distinctive application of AP(E)L, and it contrasts with the other main, instrumental, purpose of AP(E)L as part of CPD provision.

Institutions are using AP(E)L, with its promise of saving students time and money, as a 'marketing tool to increase the attractiveness of their part-time provision' (UCAS, 1996, p. 9). Part-time and vocational students represent the fastest-growing sector of HE, particularly in professions such as nursing and health-care studies, social work and management.

AP(E)L AND NEW WORK PATTERNS

Commentators and researchers on the restructuring of work (e.g. Edwards, 1993, on post-Fordism and Handy, 1990, on the creation of the 'portfolio worker') draw a picture of organizations shrinking their permanent establishments to a small nucleus of highly skilled professionals and increasingly drawing on a 'pool' of professional (and other) workers engaged on short-term and temporary contracts. In the new delayered and downsized organizations, career progression no longer lies in working one's way up the hierarchy: most professionals will have to secure their own career development, establishing their own coherent progression of work experiences and training. Increasingly, they will have to pay for it themselves too.

Many of the activities that a candidate carries out when s/he makes an application for AP(E)L involve procedures that are helpful in coping with the insecurities and unpredictability of new career patterns. These activities include:

- engaging in systematic reflection with an informed helper on what has been achieved by past experiences;
- compiling portfolio records of work histories and training courses;
- formulating training plans;
- identifying courses, work experience and qualifications that have helped achieve those plans to date;
- drawing up a career plan for the future.

That these strategies are found in AP(E)L procedures leads the UCAS document to foresee that it will have a 'key role' in relation to part-time provision and lifelong learning.

INSTRUMENTAL BENEFITS OF AP(E)L

The economic implications of lifelong learning for the 'portfolio professional' are that funding career development is increasingly left to the individual him/herself. This is why, for the individual professional (and his/her employer) AP(E)L represents such good value. HE's need to continue to find CPD part-time students has also influenced the rapid innovation of so many varieties of HE accreditation for work-based learning, e.g. having in-house training courses accredited by universities (such as happens for engineers and other Ford employees at Anglia Polytechnic University and the University of East London) and schemes where HE lecturers go into companies to teach part of professional degrees and diplomas to staff.

For all these professionals the instrumental value of AP(E)L is clear: it helps to speed up their route to higher qualifications in a very competitive job market. AP(E)L can help to raise the qualification profiles of many occupations while saving both candidates and their employers time and money.

INTRINSIC BENEFITS OF AP(E)L

There is also the intrinsic value of the period of structured reflection involved for certain groups of professionals (nursing, teaching, social work) where the model of effective professional practice sees such reflection as central to experiential learning.

Thus far, our account has dealt with political or social factors affecting the spread of AP(E)L since the 1970s. The same period has also seen an increasingly sophisticated debate about the nature of experiential learning. As more and more mature learners enter HE, so a literature has developed, drawing largely on psychology and theories of learning, to explore and explain how adults learn at work and outside classrooms. Much of this literature is by now very familiar in the field of CPD: Kolb (1984), Schon (1991), Boud, Keogh and Walker (1985), Eraut (1994).

AP(E)L AND THE HEALTH PROFESSIONS

Professional bodies such as the English National Board for Nursing, Midwifery and Health Visiting (ENB) and the Chartered Society of Physiotherapy (CSP) use the 'reflective practitioner' as the fundamental model of effective practice. These bodies have chosen portfolios as the vehicle for supporting the professionalization in their respective occupations. The above list of activities that Handy's 'portfolio worker' now needs to pursue are all included in these health professional portfolios. Completion of the portfolio demonstrates the individual's successful commitment to their own CPD. (For a detailed discussion of the principles and practice of such portfolios, see Bloor and Butterworth, 1996.)

The possibility that the individual may want to make an AP(E)L claim is built into the portfolio. Both professions are seeking to enhance the status and knowledge base of their practitioners by becoming graduate professions, and here the instrumental use of AP(E)L mentioned earlier fits with this purpose: it can help solve the structural problem set by Project 2000, i.e. the need to upgrade the qualifications of large numbers of existing nurses as new norms of initial training are set. This structural problem affects all levels: there have been huge numbers of enrolled nurses (ENs) needing conversion and RGN nurses needing to progress to graduate status (putting pressure first on diploma-level, then degree-level nursing courses). Above the level of initial training another trend in CPD is now marked: the growing prevalence (in all professions) of a master's degree as the 'qualification of choice' for the mid-career professional.

The potential importance of AP(E)L is underlined by the fact that it is a requirement for colleges wishing to be validated for the ENB Higher Award that they must have an AP(E)L system (Selway and McHale, 1994). It is also an essential component of the UKCC Standards for Post-Registration Programmes, which lead to Specialist Practitioner status. There are many examples of the successful use of AP(E)L in such professional courses to help accelerate the progress of students – the case studies in the second part of this chapter give details of three such schemes.

The second major reason for the nursing profession's acceptance of AP(E)L lies in the intellectual and academic importance of the model of reflective practice that underpins many AP(E)L procedures. Where experiential learning is accepted as equal to study-based learning, a new partnership can develop between HE and the professions for whom it provides CPD. An AP(E)L process is 'developmental' to the extent that it stresses the importance of helping candidates to reflect on their previous work experience, to see patterns of coherence and progression in their professional life and to trace the connections between their developing skills and knowledge and those that their current course will strengthen. AP(E)L, which is based on strong developmental values, fits well with the model of the reflective practitioner. (At this point it is appropriate to remove the brackets around the E for experiential, as the discussion that follows applies only to experiential learning, since assessing prior certificated learning is a simpler process: assessors only have to decide the relevance and credit value of previous qualifications or training courses.)

THE APEL PROCESS

What are the stages in the process of making an APEL claim? The discussion that follows looks at these in detail and illustrates with a fictitious (perhaps 'factitious' might be more accurate, since it's based on characteristics of candidates we have worked with) example.

Helping a student answer questions such as 'What have I learnt?', 'How did I learn it?' and 'What relevance has that learning to my academic and career plans/developing expertise?' is part of any APEL procedure, which can be summarized as the following series of initial questions:

- What past work and training experience do I have?
- What have I learned from these experiences?
- Which of this learning is relevant to this course?

The following case study demonstrates how this process may occur.

WHAT PAST WORK AND TRAINING EXPERIENCES DO I HAVE?

Sarah is a registered nurse working in an Accident and Emergency (A&E) department. She has been qualified for 5 years and recently undertook the ENB Course 199 – Accident and Emergency Nursing, which was credit-rated. Some 4 years ago she attended the ENB Course 998 – Teaching and Assessing in Clinical Practice, which was not credit-rated. Since then she has attended a range of study days related to the scope of professional practice and a workshop and conference on the management of violence and aggression in health-care settings.

Following the ENB 998 course Sarah has been able to apply learning gained on the course to develop her practice. She planned and organized a teaching programme for the department, which includes contributions from herself and other members of the multidisciplinary team.

Sarah is especially interested in promoting effective communication within the department, particularly in relation to the education of patients. She has worked with colleagues and patients to produce literature in the form of advice leaflets and educational posters for the department.

Sarah has also developed her knowledge and understanding of factors giving rise to violence and aggression in A&E. She has read extensively following the workshop and attended other departments to discuss how they manage the environment to reduce the incidence of violence and aggression. Sarah has subsequently reviewed working practices within the department and negotiated certain changes to enhance communication between staff and clients. She was instrumental in producing a standard for dealing with violent incidents in the department. Colleagues in the department recognize her expertise and seek her advice on matters relating to aggression management. As a result of this she has produced a resource/teaching package on managing violence and aggression for staff and students working in the A&E department.

Sarah has applied the general learning gained on the continuing education programmes and from her years of working in accident and emergency nursing and developed it in relation to specific areas of her practice. It is now her intention to complete a degree in clinical practice, but she has insufficient credit at level 2. Sarah has spent considerable time researching and developing the various initiatives and believes that the experiential learning outlined is substantial enough for her to make a claim for APEL.

WHAT HAVE I LEARNED FROM THESE EXPERIENCES?

At this stage Sarah finds it difficult to articulate the learning outcomes precisely but is able to identify her achievements and areas of expertise in general terms. She makes notes about the activities in which she has been involved within the department:

- 'I have discussed aspects of practice with colleagues and identified the topics to include in a teaching programme within the A&E department. I also organize and participate in the teaching programme to meet those needs and encourage colleagues to be involved.
- 'I have gathered and read information about violence and aggression and participated in writing a standard to deal with violent and aggressive situations.
- 'I have produced a resource package about management of violence and aggression in A&E.
- 'I am often asked to give advice on matters relating to violence and aggression management in A&E.
- 'I have reviewed discharge information for clients and produced advisory leaflets.'

WHICH OF THIS LEARNING IS RELEVANT TO THIS COURSE?

Sarah reads the course outcomes and the level 2 criteria and believes that her learning matches certain areas of the curriculum. She decides that she wishes to proceed with an APEL claim. She discusses this with the course leader, who advises her about the process and arranges for her to meet the APEL coordinator, who confirms that the claim is substantial enough to proceed.

Sarah now has access to help and advice from an APEL advisor through workshops and individual tutorials.

Many schemes emphasize the importance of tutorial support (or appropriate materials) early in the stages of the APEL claim, when the candidate is helped to consider these questions.

Candidates do not find it easy to move from a factual, descriptive work/training record to an identification of the learning involved, in terms of increased skills and knowledge.

The next stage of the process requires that their learning be expressed in a form that can be matched with course objectives, usually in the form of learning outcomes.

These can be written by the candidate or selected from course literature. The questions at this stage are:

- Which course outcomes can I claim to have already achieved?
- How can I 'prove' that I have achieved them (i.e. what evidence and testimonials can I provide that will support my claim)?

Sarah's claim will be for general credit, i.e. against the overall outcomes of the programme rather than specified unit outcomes.

WHICH OF THE COURSE OUTCOMES CAN I CLAIM TO HAVE ALREADY ACHIEVED?

With the help of her advisor Sarah reflects upon her experiences and the general learning statements she made. She is now able to identify specific outcomes from these experiences and to match them to the level 2 course outcomes more precisely. In achieving this the advisor asks Sarah a range of questions such as 'What prompted you to do that?', 'How did you go about that?', 'Why do you think that was successful?'. This assists her in clarifying the learning and skills that she has acquired.

The outcomes of the programme state the learning in general terms and Sarah writes her own outcomes that fulfil this.

One outcome is as follows: 'Demonstrate the ability to facilitate and assess both professional and developmental needs of those for whom responsible and act as a role model of professional practice'.

Sarah is able to:

- identify the development needs of staff and implement strategies to meet these needs;
- act as a role model in the clinical area, in relation to the facilitation of learning for clients and colleagues;
- research and design teaching materials for clients and colleagues.

Another outcome states: 'Demonstrate the ability to evaluate the quality of care delivered within the practice setting'.

Sarah is able to:

- discuss the need for standards in nursing and use an established format to design standard statements;
- work as an effective multiagency team member and promote cooperation in the delivery of quality health care.

HOW CAN I PROVE THAT I HAVE ACHIEVED THEM? WHAT EVIDENCE DO I HAVE?

Sarah collects a range of direct evidence in support of her claim, materials such as teaching plans, the resource package, advice leaflets and protocols for dealing with violent or potentially violent situations. Her manager also agrees to provide further indirect evidence in the form of a written statement regarding her role as advisor within the department.

With guidance from her advisor Sarah then writes a supportive account of how these experiences have developed her both personally and professionally. This includes analysing her practice, demonstrating an understanding of relevant theoretical concepts and the way literature and research have influenced her learning.

Finally Sarah collates all the evidence of her learning and organizes the information in her file according to the instructions she has received.

Her portfolio is now complete and can be submitted for assessment.

Documentary proof and evidence of learning provide material that allows some objective assessment to take place, judging the evidence of experiential learning by the standards used to assess study-based learning. Candidates may be asked to produce some kind of supporting statement or commentary, either in the form of writing or during the course of an assessment interview.

Asking APEL candidates to reflect on their past learning and to identify its links to present study encourages them to conceptualize their practice to match areas of current research and professional debate, and helps them establish the relevance of current theoretical debate to their own practice. Such activities are at the heart of the concept of reflective practice, though there are differences in the importance that assessors place on candidates showing knowledge of formal, published theory in their accounts.

CASE STUDIES OF CURRENT AP(E)L PRACTICE

It is useful at this point to consider the following case studies, which illustrate the way in which three individual institutions within the UK are implementing the AP(E)L process. (For a comparison of different approaches to APEL in a sample of current schemes, including nursing courses, see Butterworth and McKelvey, 1997.)

These approaches have common features in that they are drawn from healthcare education and have been operating for a minimum of 3 years. The first example is taken from a new university and features a model of APEL incorporated within a BSc (Hons) Physiotherapy distance learning programme, which is one of a suite of programmes designed to enable traditionally trained health professionals to develop professionally and gain academic awards.

The second example concerns APEL within a credit scheme for qualified nurses and midwives entering diploma and degree programmes linked to professional awards within a traditional university.

The third illustrates the APEL process in a traditional university where a collaborative approach across a range of health-care courses exists. Students achieve accreditation by undertaking a dedicated APEL unit.

Within the text the term 'level' refers to Credit Accumulation and Transfer Scheme (CATS) levels 1, 2 and3.

- Level 1 – 120 credits – Certificate
- Level 2 – 120 credits – Diploma
- Level 3 – 120 credits – Degree.

APEL at a distance: distance learning top-up degree for diplomate physiotherapists

Pre-course information

Information regarding AP(E)L within the university is detailed in the prospectus. The specific course information sent to students outlines the role of AP(E)L within the programme and how it may be achieved.

The programme seeks to recognize the wealth of prior learning that the student has and to enable them to top up their current award to degree level by achieving 120 credits at level 3. The volume of credit that can be awarded against this programme via AP(E)L is 50%.

Access

Participants enter the programme with 240 credits at level 2 in respect of their diploma or graduate diploma in physiotherapy.

The 120 credits at level 3 required are achieved through the process of accreditation of prior experiential learning [APEL] and/or accreditation of prior certificated learning [APL] to a maximum of 60 credits and a compulsory research component of 60 credits. This enables the student to design a flexible and individualized programme that takes advantage of both professional and academic development. The Research Preparation and Research Project units are designed to be the synoptic phase of the programme, providing coherence and progression.

The credit for APL, i.e. certificated learning, is awarded as part of the Chartered Society of Physiotherapists – Strategy for Continuing Professional Development (formerly Physiotherapy Access to Continuing Education programme – PACE). Within this framework the Chartered Society and the University of Greenwich recognize and confer a credit rating on numerous professional development courses that are offered outside the higher education sector.

For those students making an APEL claim this commences upon access to the programme. The students provide a statement of intent, which includes details of the areas of experience for which they intend to develop a claim for APEL.

Guidance

Each student is then allocated an advisor to assist them in the process of preparing a portfolio of prior experiential learning. A guidance workbook is also sent to the student. This contains general information about APEL and provides specific detail regarding the production of the portfolio of evidence. Relevant examples are cited and the student is encouraged to work through the various exercises designed to develop his/her reflective skills.

Access to 6 hours of tutorial support is provided by a range of methods including telephone, computer-mediated communication and correspondence. Students opt for one or more approaches as need dictates. The role of the advisor is to facilitate the process of development and assist the student in the articulation of learning that has taken place.

Assessment

Until this stage of the process the approach has been unique to this programme of study in order to meet the student's very specific requirements. At the assessment phase the process dovetails with the approach taken within the university credit scheme. The completed portfolio is submitted for assessment and is reviewed for relevance, sufficiency, currency and level by a specialist/physiotherapist who will not have played any role in the facilitation of the student.

The portfolio is then moderated by a second lecturer, ideally a physiotherapy lecturer with APEL experience. It is scrutinized in the same way as any other piece of academic work to ensure consistency in the award of amount and level of credit.

Portfolios are also subject to scrutiny by an external examiner and agreed by an APL monitoring committee before being ratified by the Board of Examiners.

The student is then notified of the credit awarded and it is recorded on the student profile within the university database.

Percentage of students who undertake AP(E)L

Of the students accessing the pathway 100% will make an APL claim and 70% an APEL claim.

Costing

The cost is £70 per 10 credits claimed, which is equivalent to approximately one third of the course cost.

Key features of this approach

This approach to APEL offers the student increased flexibility within his/her programme of study. It facilitates the student's ability to maximize prior learning whether certificated or experiential. Some systems, while allowing reasonable percentages of APL against an award, impose ceilings on the amounts of APEL that can be obtained within the overall percentage. This model recognizes that many practitioners have advanced their practice over a number of years by gaining experience in very specialized areas of practice for which no formal training was offered. Often these practitioners are pioneering developments in practice within the area of specialism; this requires them to learn varied and complex skills. The total flexibility within the AP(E)L allowance creates an opportunity for such practitioners to achieve full recognition of their learning from experience and upholds the principle of achieving greater access.

The student making the claim will be required to identify practice-based learning and provide current evidence of this in a sufficiently focused manner to allow comparison against level 3 academic criteria. This will be a reasonable task for a large section of the professionals accessing the programme but it will also be attracting a group who have not undertaken academic study for a long time and who may not have the range of academic skills required to express their learning sufficiently well to warrant credit at degree level. Developing these skills in isolation from other students can be very daunting, especially if the practitioner has not studied for some time.

Group tutorials or a mixture of individual and group tutorials are approaches favoured by many institutions, as students may gain considerable benefit from working alongside others who are aiming for similar goals (Simosko, 1991). While this distance approach ensures the student has access to appropriate support and advice to assist in the process, it does not provide the student with the opportunity to work alongside others making a learning claim.

AP(E)L within one traditional university: a credit scheme for qualified nurses and midwives entering diploma and degree programmes linked to professional awards

Pre-course information

Information regarding the use of AP(E)L within the university is detailed quite extensively in the prospectus. Further information is provided in a handbook on credit accumulation and profiling that is given to students prior to entering the programme of study.

It is important to note that qualified nurses and midwives have advanced standing for level 1: 120 credits by virtue of their first-level qualification. The volume of credit that can be awarded against the courses in the credit scheme is 50% at diploma level and a maximum of 15 credits at level 3.

Access

Access to a programme of study within this scheme is by application and interview.

First-level and some second-level nurses undertaking diploma and degree
awards in nursing/midwifery can gain exemption from level 1 study through the
interview process; however, it is possible to access the scheme without interview
and undertake a free-standing course

All claims for AP(E)L level 2 exemption require the production of a profile.

Those students with prior certificated learning at level 2 are required to produce
a profile that contains copies of their certificates and a statement in support of their
claim, rather than the more in-depth profile required for APEL claims.

Guidance

Potential AP(E)L candidates are advised to attend one of the 16 AP(E)L workshops that are offered annually. The purpose of this 1-day workshop is to provide
information about AP(E)L in general and guidance on the protocol for making a
claim within a specific programme of study. The day is supported by up to three
tutors, who participate in small group facilitation and individual support for those
wishing to make a claim. This activity is also used for staff development as it provides the opportunity for staff new to the AP(E)L process to develop their skills
with support and guidance from colleagues.

Students making a claim are required to complete an AP(E)L claim form.
Instruction and assistance are given regarding the completion of this form and
sometimes this involves giving career advice. Discussion occurs regarding the presentation of the profile and a handbook is provided in support of this. At the end
of the day, if the student decides to make a claim s/he is expected to produce an
action plan for the process. Students are required to make their claims against
specific modules/courses within a designated pathway rather than against the overall pathway.

Additional support in the preparation of the claim is available following the
workshop, according to need. It is recognized that some students do require considerable assistance in preparing a claim; however, the time a student may demand
of the tutor is unspecified. Extra guidance is generally given by the course leader
or students may seek assistance from another tutor who is involved in the accreditation process. This support is recorded as *ad hoc* activity in order that it can be
estimated and charged to the student's employing trust.

Assessment

Completed profiles are submitted to the APL coordinator, who distributes to designated assessors. The assessor will be a contributing lecturer on the programme
of study against which the student is making a claim and will not normally have

been involved to any great extent in the facilitation of the student. All profiles are assessed by two lecturers, the second assessor being another subject specialist or the course leader.

The profile is then presented for moderation and ratification to a divisional accreditation panel, who agree credit awarded. This panel comprises academic staff from the university Department of Nursing Studies and from the Division of Nursing and Midwifery. The student is notified of credit awarded and it is recorded on the student profile within the university database.

Percentage of students undertaking AP(E)L

Of the 1000 students accessing the scheme approximately 20% will make an APL claim against an award, a small number of whom will make an APEL claim.

Costings

Where a pre-existing contract with a trust exists for postregistration students the charge for AP(E)L is charged as one study day from the trust allocation of training days. For other students the fee is £45.

Key features of this approach

A positive aspect of this approach is the frequency with which the potential student can gain access to advice and support about the AP(E)L process from tutorial staff.

The cost is not prohibitive, even for those students who will not receive funding and may have to pay themselves. Very clear messages are being sent to students regarding the commitment to AP(E)L within this particular scheme. Such an approach should serve to create a greater number of APEL claims than are currently being made. This may be indicative of the anxieties many students have in relation to reflective skills. Experience of such students indicates that many prefer to undertake a taught unit rather than grapple with the concepts of reflection; some find the process emotionally draining and perceive it as a considerable amount of effort for what may in the end be only a small amount of credit.

In this institution, as in many nationally, it is nursing and the health-related courses that are forging ahead with the process of AP(E)L. Success lies in convincing the traditional areas of the university, where a more cautious approach is taken.

AP(E)L within a collaborative health scheme in a traditional university

Pre-course information

Currently the university prospectus does not contain specific information regarding AP(E)L. However, the pre-course information sent to students undertaking health courses contains details regarding the availability of AP(E)L within the programmes of study. Student handbooks also contain information about making an AP(E)L claim.

Students can gain information about the health courses from an Access, Guidance and Accreditation Unit that has recently been established. Students are referred to the Academic Coordinator, who provides specific help and advice on an individual basis. Students seeking this advice are requested to complete a form detailing their personal and professional development needs. This provides a focus for discussion and assists the student in clarifying his/her requirements. During this meeting a programme of study may be developed and the student can discuss AP(E)L opportunities if this is appropriate. The volume of credit which can be awarded against a programme of study within the health scheme is 50%.

Access

Those students who wish to make a straightforward APL claim against their chosen award will be referred to the appropriate admissions tutor, who will advise them. They are required to complete a pro-forma detailing courses undertaken and to provide a supporting statement detailing how this learning contributes to their chosen programme of study. However, the scheme is moving towards a tariff approach for APL.

If a student wishes to make a claim for his/her experiential learning the academic coordinator will advise him/her. Once it is established that the student has substantial relevant experience to make a claim s/he is registered to undertake the Accreditation and Programme Planning Unit.

Guidance

A new system of guidance has recently been introduced as part of the role of the Access Guidance and Accreditation Unit. Currently it is compulsory for any student who wishes to make an APEL claim to undertake the Accreditation and Programme Planning Unit – a 10 credit level 2 unit. Students who make a successful claim, regardless of level and amount, are awarded a further 10 level 2 credits in recognition of the skills acquired in extrapolating evidence and producing the portfolio.

The unit comprises 15 hours of advice and guidance in a classroom setting. Information is given concerning credit schemes and the AP(E)L process, programme structure and formulating an individual programme of study. The group also explores reflective practice and personal and professional development. Through a series of group and individual tutorials the student is assisted in systematic reflection on experience and the identification of learning. The group support is provided by the academic coordinator, who coopts relevant specialist teachers to assist in the process as necessary. A further 4 hours of individual tutorial guidance is available to each student, although the uptake will vary according to student needs. At the end of the unit the student produces a personal portfolio of learning, which contains specific claims against particular module[s] outcomes from a programme of study rather than against the programme in general.

Assessment

The completed portfolio is submitted to the admissions tutor, who makes the initial assessment and agrees the credit rating. This tutor will not have been involved in advising the student when preparing the portfolio. An APL working group has been established within the school whose function is to scrutinize the portfolio and endorse the decision of the admissions tutor. Further moderation is undertaken by the external examiner at the appropriate board of examiners. The student is notified of credit awarded and a record of achievement is entered in the student's record.

Percentage of students undertaking AP(E)L

Approximately 1000 students access the health courses and of this number approximately 20% will make an APL claim. APEL claims are significantly lower, approximately 20 claims being made annually. The previous lack of information available to students and the lack of expertise in advising students are believed to account for this. It is anticipated that the numbers will increase substantially with the implementation of the dedicated APEL unit and the growth of the collaborative scheme to include the professions allied to medicine.

Costings

The cost for the APEL unit is the same as the module cost, which is £150. This fee is separate from the course cost and is the responsibility of the individual making the application.

Key features of this approach

A significant feature of this approach is the opportunity for the student to gain credit for the developmental aspects of making an APEL claim; many students acknowledge that considerable personal and professional growth occurs from this process. Another advantage of offering the APEL process within a unit structure is that it gives APEL status alongside other academic units. Students have the opportunity to gain from both the group and individual facilitation and thus to maximize learning. It also provides the opportunity for the facilitators to create an environment that is conducive to reflection, which may not be as readily achievable in other approaches. The student is consistently exposed to the same lecturers and colleagues over a period of time and with the appropriate support it is more likely that a relationship of trust will develop, which enhances a developmental model of APEL.

A possible issue for concern might be that the overall process is labour-intensive. This highly student-centred approach with initial pre-course advice and guidance along with diagnostic and developmental work does have significant resource implications, particularly if the demand for APEL increases. However, it is possible that this is a highly effective use of resources: those involved report an increased retention rate within the programmes of study, which may well be attributed to the considerable time spent in pre-course developmental work.

The UCAS survey (1996) usefully summarizes the issues that have to be addressed by those setting up or monitoring their own APEL procedures. In the final section we discuss those issues and relate them to other current debate about aspects of APEL practice in higher education.

CRITICAL ISSUES AS APEL PRACTICE DEVELOPS

General or Specific credit?

It seems more common for AP(E)L candidates to claim for specific credit (matching their own learning against published module or unit outcomes) than for general credit. This is probably because few courses have published outcomes that are at the level of the overall award, in addition to outcomes at module or unit level. The BSc (Hons) Physiotherapy Studies, previously mentioned, has stated overall aims and outcomes against which the student must make his/her learning claim.

An example of one overarching outcome is as follows: the practitioner will be able to 'demonstrate an ability to reflect in and on practice and through this process, enhance their professional development'.

The outcome is sufficiently flexible for students to determine the areas of practice where they have acquired knowledge and skills, which will form the focus of the claim. They may be able to articulate learning across a range of activities, e.g. management, health promotion, practical skills, which together formulate significant development and advances in their overall professional practice but which would not meet specific outcomes of an individual unit. The learning identified must also comply with the stated assessment criteria and the definition of level 3 educational activity within the scheme.

Assessing specific credit may be simpler (it can be done by module subject specialists) but it may have disadvantages for some candidates if it is the only option offered to them. A candidate who has to match module outcomes may have to 'narrow' their experiential learning to fit subject- or discipline-based outcomes. Candidates may give greater priority to 'finding the outcome to match' than to reflecting on their past experience in order to distinguish their own outcomes.

Balancing 'accessible' AP(E)L against quality assurance demands

It is important to design an AP(E)L procedure that does not make candidates jump through more hoops than students gaining credit by the normal study route. Many staff keen to introduce AP(E)L, in many different HE systems, report the suspicions of colleagues who see it as a development that will dilute standards. AP(E)L practitioners also comment on the opposite dangers: that over-rigorous procedures will only benefit the already skilled student rather than genuinely open up access. Clearly there are very important issues at stake here: AP(E)L portfolios must be subject to the same monitoring and moderation procedures as other formally assessed work.

Staff unused to dealing with portfolios or assessing practical, experiential learning may need staff development. Where portfolios may be assessed by different subject specialists, they must share common assessment criteria. Whatever format is adopted for the portfolio, compiling it should not demand more study, academic or organizational skills from the candidate than other coursework. Consideration must be given to the fact that, by its nature, an APEL claim is often the first piece of formally assessed work a student does on a programme: it should not be too intimidating, though it should demonstrate a level of intellectual rigour appropriate for the programme.

Charging for APEL

Schemes vary both in how they charge candidates for APEL and how they assess their own costs. Guidance and support for candidates, particularly in the early stages, are important. Providing this through face-to-face tutoring (whether individually or for groups of candidates) may be the most expensive method in terms of resources: some schemes have introduced distance materials (Butterworth and Edwards, 1993) or developed software to provide IT support. Candidates may pay for APEL at the price of a course module or unit, they may pay a fee that covers the tutoring and a separate fee for assessment or the price may vary according to the amount of credit received. In many schemes, the initial information and guidance is provided free, and only candidates who successfully submit claims pay a fee. The UCAS document (1996) gives examples of the different practices of charging candidates.

Confidentiality and power

A crucial issue is the nature of the advisory support provided. It is not easy to develop a cost-effective APEL process that offers enough of the right kind of support. Evaluation of schemes (see, for example, Butterworth and Edwards, 1993) shows that candidates may need a lot of information, guidance and support in the early stages, and the advisor's role can be complex and significant. At later stages, as candidates reflect on their past experience, the advisor may play a key role in helping them perceive and articulate connections between their own past learning and the way such professional areas are conceptualized in the programme.

This is a subtle and complex area. Increasingly, research and writers on adult learning are expressing concern about the potential intrusiveness of using personal reflection for formal assessment. (A particularly useful exploration of this issue in APEL is in Fraser, 1995.) There are obvious concerns about confidentiality: professionals do not feel absolutely free to write about past errors or crises (often the events we learn most from), their own or their colleagues' or manager's, in a document that will be formally assessed in the public domain. This is a sensitive issue relevant to the assessment of any kind of portfolio that asks for personal responses to professional issues (Bloor and Butterworth, 1996). Because the material can be more personal than that required for a formal essay, the candidate's vulnerability is correspondingly heightened. The advisor needs to be very aware of appropriate boundaries here, and to negotiate these with the candidate. When the programme is part of CPD, such assessments are also part of career advancement and the assessor's power is correspondingly augmented.

Practical issues follow from these concerns: practitioners continue to support the separation of the role of advisor and assessor – the same individual should not perform both functions for a candidate. A vulnerable (or dishonest) candidate may try to inflate the value of his/her past experience – the assessment procedures for judging evidence as sufficient and authentic, and for moderating those decisions, need to be as rigorous as possible.

FUTURE DEVELOPMENT OF AP(E)L

The review of international developments in the early part of this chapter established the key role that AP(E)L has to play in policies for lifelong learning. Much innovative practice is developing in higher education in the UK, and AP(E)L can make a significant contribution to professional training and development in the health professions. The discussion of critical areas in the practice of AP(E)L is part of a continuing debate that features strongly in the papers of two national conferences on the practice of AP(E)L in HE (SEEC, 1996; Bailey and O'Hagan, 1997). It will be interesting to see, as practice spreads, how far the 'founding principles' of AP(E)L – of facilitating access and progression – are delivered or transformed by its wider implementation.

ACKNOWLEDGEMENTS

The authors would like to thank all colleagues who have contributed materials for the case studies within this chapter; in particular staff within the School of Health, University of Greenwich and the Nursing and Midwifery Division, King's College, London.

REFERENCES

Bailey, S. and O'Hagan, C. (eds) (1997) *Accrediting Prior Learning in Higher Education: A Northern Ireland Perspective*, University of Ulster, Belfast.

Barkatoolah, A. (1997) From competence audit to APL: the French experience of APL in higher education, in *Accrediting Prior Learning in Higher Education: A Northern Ireland Perspective*, (eds Bailey, S. and O'Hagan, C.), University of Ulster, Belfast.

Barnett, R. (1990) *The Idea of Higher Education*, Society for Research into Higher Education/Open University Press, Milton Keynes.

Bloor, M. and Butterworth, C. (1996) The portfolio approach to professional development, in *The Professional FE Teacher: Staff Development and Training in the Corporate FE College*, (ed. J. Robson), Avebury, Aldershot.

Boud, D., Keogh, R. and Walker, D. (1985) *Reflection: Turning Experience into Learning*, Kogan Page, London.

Butterworth, C. and Edwards, R. (1993) Accrediting prior learning at a distance. *Open Learning*, **8**(3).

Butterworth, C. and McKelvey, C. (1997) A study of APEL in four universities. *Journal of Access Studies*, **12**(2), 153–175.

CNAA (1988) The assessment of prior experiential learning. *CNAA Development Services Publication 17*, Council for National Academic Awards, London.

Cohen, R., Flowers, R., McDonald, R. and Schaafsma, H. (1993) *Learning From Experience Counts. Recognition of Prior Learning in Australian Universities*. University of Technology, Sydney, NSW.

Edwards, R. (1993) The inevitable future? Post-Fordism in work and learning, in *Adult Learners, Education and Training*, (eds R. Edwards, S. Sieminski and D. Zeldin), Routledge/Open University, London.

Eraut, M. (1994) *Developing Professional Knowledge and Competence*, Falmer Press, London.

Fraser, W. (1995) *Learning from Experience: Empowerment or Incorporation?* National Institute for Adult and Continuing Education, Leicester.

Handy, C. (1990) *The Age of Unreason*, Arrow Books, London.

Harre Hindmarsh, J. (1992) Recognition of prior learning in a New Zealand University: an exploratory study. *New Zealand Journal of Adult Learning*, **20**(2).

Hornblow, D. (1995) Recognition of Prior Learning: a mix of accessibility, quality and economic viability, in *Proceedings of the RPL Institute*, RPL Services, Wellington.

Kolb, D. (1984) *Experiential Learning*, Prentice-Hall, London.

Schon, D. (1991) *The Reflective Practitioner*, Avebury, Aldershot.

SEEC (1995) AP(E)L: a quality code for AP(E)L: *Issues for Managers and Practitioners*, in *Proceedings of the SEEC National Conference*, South East England Consortium for Credit Accumulation and Transfer, Anglia Polytechnic University, Brentwood.

Selway, I. and McHale, C. (1994) Integrating professional education and training into higher education award structures using the accreditation of prior learning. *Journal of Access Studies*, **9**(1).

Simosko, S. (1991) *APL: A Practical Guide for Professionals*, Kogan Page, London.

Stock, A. (1996) Lifelong Learning: thirty years of educational change, in *The Learning Society*, (eds P. Raggatt, R. Edwards and N. Small), Routledge/Open University, London.

UCAS (1996) *Accreditation of Prior Learning: Briefing for Higher Education*, Universities and Colleges Admissions Service, Cheltenham.

UDACE (1991) *What can Graduates Do? A Consultative Paper*, Unit for the Development of Adult and Continuing Education, Leicester.

<table>
<tr><td>12</td><td># Nursing informatics</td></tr>
</table>

12	# Nursing informatics

Liz Stubbings and Lynn Woodward

BACKGROUND

The evolution of nursing informatics within the UK has been insidious in nature and has encompassed many of the aspects of the technological nature of nursing. Within the health-care environment practitioners have had varying degrees of exposure to the technological innovations in clinical practice that have developed over recent years.

The implementation of technology and information systems has been generally fragmented across the UK health service. This in part was due to the lack of any cohesive NHS strategy for technology prior to the late 1980s, and in part to the rate at which the use of technology developed and was incorporated into practice in certain parts of the health service (e.g. laboratory services, finance department). Nursing has been isolated in many areas of practice from the technological developments and academic debate surrounding informatics, the main discussions stemming from North America and Scandinavia.

The need for nursing to have a heightened awareness of informatics has evolved following statutory changes in health-care practice and management. The publication of the NHS strategy for information management and technology (NHSME, 1992) and subsequent guidelines for the management of data have given clarification to the professions. The recognition of specific professional needs in relation to technology pertaining to patient care and information management has been addressed by professional bodies. It is now advocated by the National Boards for Nursing and Midwifery that technology is incorporated into preregistration curricula. This is not interpreted as teaching just 'hands on' computing skills, but also incorporates the skills relating to information management and application of technology in clinical practice as this directly impacts upon patient care and the profession.

In order for technology to impact upon future evidence-based practice it is vital that the student develops the necessary knowledge, skills and attitudes. This will provide a more integrated approach to informatics to mirror the multifaceted milieu that the learner encounters within many diverse clinical environments. Such attributes should combine with nursing theory for implementation in practice. The principles underpinning this philosophy are based on the need to create lifelong learners (ENB, 1995) and the Information Management Group's strategic statement (NHSME, 1994).

This enables progression and the marrying of nursing knowledge with technology so that this concept is viewed as whole and not as separate entities.

DEFINITION

The term 'nursing informatics' itself is interpreted differently by practitioners in different fields and hence authors of the subject have had difficulty in defining the term with any consistency. This is in part because of the different professional viewpoints, the different information needs of those within the professions and indeed the eclectic nature of nursing itself.

Leeder (1991) defines nursing informatics as:

the use of nursing science, computer science and information science in nursing processes for patient/client care which provides data, information and knowledge to the individual and the organization in such a way as to change/influence society while protecting the individual and achieving health for all.

This definition highlights for practitioners a number of aims of nursing informatics, the main aim being a combination of computer science and nursing knowledge in order to create and integrate meaningful information that can be accessed by those in nursing and allied professions, thus stressing that nursing science is based on professional judgement and informed decision-making and is not just a series of tasks. Nursing informatics is also an efficient vehicle for presenting to practitioners networks for communication, ongoing education and research in order to promote quality practice. It also provides practitioners with an effective management medium within health care, with the ultimate aim of enhancing the health of society.

The efficacy of nursing informatics is interdependent with the individual's receptiveness and the effective functioning of the technology itself. Informatics can be viewed as a powerful tool in respect of the potential information that can be extracted and used to influence decisions across the health spectrum.

INFORMATICS IN PRACTICE

Most practitioners have initially encountered nursing informatics within the practice environment where it is incorporated as part of the wider remit of health informatics within the health-care setting. Health-care systems, such as hospital information support systems (HISS), midwifery or community information systems, have developed to incorporate nursing components; in other areas stand-alone nursing systems operate that do not integrate information with other health-care disciplines. The information that nurses are required to input into a system varies according to the nature of work and the capability of the system in operation. In the main, nursing staff are responsible for the inputting of a client's demographic details, assessment data and the subsequent generation of a plan of care. Within existing midwifery systems routine data that is required legally, such as birth notifications, are component parts. All information systems serve practitioners as a communication tool within their own discipline and integrated systems provide the means for interdisciplinary communication. The wider remit of nursing systems can also accommodate nursing databases to store protocols and a library of client information to facilitate research and audit, patient dependency calculation, internal ordering facilities, staff rostering and budgeting tools that act as decision support mechanisms.

It is of paramount importance that a system ensures that the pragmatic information needs of the profession and the organization in which professionals operate are met. The ability of nursing informatics to provide practitioners with the necessary framework for the storage of applicable data and the subsequent extraction of useful information depends upon the attitudes, knowledge and skills of both practitioners and those responsible for the overseeing of system support within the organization.

ATTITUDES

Those involved in the initial procurement of the system must acknowledge, and not assume, the needs of practitioners and provide adequate functions for the inputting and retrieval of useful nursing data. Therefore, the employer must actively involve those nursing staff who will be main users in the selection of the system and the subsequent design of the nursing modules. Without this collaboration the process of installing an information system becomes more of an imposition upon the profession than an integrated, needs-based approach.

In practice the rapid momentum for information acquisition to manage and resource health care within the internal market arena, as well as to provide compulsory data at both a local and national level, has resulted in health-care information systems that are highly management-focused. This aspect has been combated by medical staff in some areas that have an integrated system, resulting in a more medical orientation to the functions available. Consequently, nursing components and functions are often omitted or overlooked as other disciplines lack awareness of what is essential to nursing.

At this juncture many practitioners feel that it is either a fruitless task to challenge the choice within the current organizational culture or do not feel satisfactorily knowledgeable or confident to articulate their concerns. This attitude, if left unaddressed, means in practice that neither the practitioner or the employer gains the maximum potential from the system. As a result many practitioners, who generate the bulk of the information, perceive that there are few benefits from a nursing or health information system that directly impact upon improving client care or the profession as a whole.

In practice, many health-care and nursing information systems are 'sold' to nursing staff on the premise that they can built upon them to form a comprehensive nursing informatics package that offers a whole gamut of tools promising to make the job easier. It is vital to the organization that nursing staff are in favour and well informed of the benefits of the system, as in practice they are responsible for the bulk of main data entry onto any system. In reality, however, the positive attributes for nursing that the system was sold upon do not always materialize in the practice environment because of incompatibilities with existing systems (e.g. patient administration systems) or lack of resources. This results in a general anticlimactic air towards the exercise as practitioners question what they actually get from the system in return for their high input.

This attitude toward nursing informatics is further compounded by the lack of access for many practitioners to the whole information picture within an organization. Limiting access to some areas is a necessity in order to comply with the Data Protection Act (1984), to protect client confidentiality and ensure that sensitive organizational information is not disclosed to competitors. Presently, accessing the relevant data and assimilating this into meaningful information that can be presented to practitioners to aid reflection upon current practice is the domain of a few, usually senior practitioners, often in a management capacity. Information gained from this source is often shrouded in suspicion and there is a prevailing lack of ownership of such material by those who most frequently use the system for data entry. In practice this often means that practitioners pay lip service to a system, inputting the minimum data required and seldom seeking to evaluate information from the system as a whole.

Such resistance in areas of the profession with regard to data collection and documentation is historically familiar. The generation of client documentation, whether manually or electronically, is often perceived as being a secondary task within the profession: the nature of nursing is to concentrate on direct care giving and not the production of written material. The need to emphasize to practitioners that client documentation is an integral part of the care process resulted in the publication of guidelines by the professional body (UKCC, 1993), Guidelines for Practice (UKCC, 1996) and the incorporation of nursing informatics into the pre-registration curriculum.

Other negative aspects are attributed to the introduction of informatics within the workplace, although when examined these are secondary effects of a changing organizational culture rather than the direct result of the system itself. Nursing staff often view the rise in paperwork, reduction in clerical support and technical involvement with IT equipment as yet another imposition of the system. In reality this is a result of inadequate support mechanisms and the ineffectiveness of nursing management to intervene and clearly delineate what tasks are nursing and which are not. This problem again is historical in nursing, the presumption being that as the prime care providers nursing staff are responsible for the overall coordination of client care and the systems that support it. In order to break away from this cycle of lack of professional self-esteem and empower practitioners there must be a change in the culture of the profession as a whole. Nursing informatics needs to be viewed as a tool to be manipulated for the benefit of the practitioner and the future of evidence-based care.

KNOWLEDGE

Many benefits for the profession and subsequent impact upon direct client care can be derived through using nursing informatics as a vehicle for learning. This medium can be capitalized upon by employers, educationalists and practitioners alike to ensure that the profession shares, develops and harnesses its knowledge base in order to progressively enhance clinical practice. However, in order to do so the profession needs to identify exactly what knowledge and nursing skills are required.

The introduction of nursing systems has emphasized to practitioners both the volume and depth of information required to maintain an accurate plan of client care. Indeed, this is not a new requirement due to the introduction of a nursing system but rather a highlighting of the inherent deficiencies of manual documentation. Insight on the part of the practitioner that such deficiencies need to be addressed in all systems of care documentation can be promoted by extending particular areas of nursing knowledge. Traditionally, the knowledge underpinning the prescription of client care has been gained through a theoretically focused nursing model and nursing process approach. The clinical skills that underpin the assessment process have not been given so much attention in practice. The result of this is a theory/practice divide that often manifests itself in superficial, irrelevant and inconsistent client care planning data.

In order to address this problem and ensure that relevant client data is captured, practitioners need to realize what data is important and what information can assist them in planning comprehensive client care. This area needs to be focused upon by employers and educationalists who have both knowledge and practical application. Regular auditing of electronically generated care plans can detect specific problems within the documentation process and deficits addressed through staff education or clinical supervision programmes. A general awareness that higher levels of assessment skills can be learned and put into practice also needs to be addressed by the profession in order to improve practice – moving it away from a intuitive base to one of a more measurable, empirical nature.

The broader remit of nursing informatics knowledge can enhance the practitioner's position in the selection of systems locally by empowering him/her to articulate his/her needs. This promotes both insight and analytical skills. Enabling practitioners to expand their knowledge and become informed has a percolating effect upon other staff and learners within the workplace. Common complaints regarding informatics, such as the nursing model employed, lack of individualization within the planning process and the apparently greater time demands upon nursing staff, can often be allayed or solved by knowledgeable peers, which is less of an imposition upon the staff concerned than if solutions are seen as emanating from a line manager.

The introduction of PREPP has highlighted the importance of continuing education within the profession but practitioners need to realize that alternative styles of learning exist beyond the more traditional methods. Employers and educationalists also need to heighten awareness and explore areas of nursing informatics that can facilitate ongoing learning for practitioners. The subject matter that nurses choose to study to remain updated in practice also needs to be reassessed. Traditionally, areas of skills-based practical nursing development have been popular within the continuing education sphere as they are construed as having a direct and measurable impact upon 'hands on' client care by practitioners. Educational institutions are also guaranteed a market in this area because of their popularity and the fact that the classroom method of delivery is cost-effective. However, other subject matter and modes of delivery need to be explored in order to offer the profession flexible and alternative learning. The development of informatics-based learning packages or tools may appear time-consuming, requiring financial investment and innovation from skilled nurse educationalists; production has therefore been relatively small, on a local basis and dependent upon market forces.

Within clinical and education environments there often exists a systems incompatibility that does not allow the practitioner to access many programs or databases. To date most nursing and HISS systems operate DOS-based packages on hardware that cannot support the Windows-based applications now being introduced into the health-care market. Therefore, access to communication networks such as the NHSWEB and Internet databases is restricted and dependent upon a PC with a connection to the 'outside' being available for practitioners' use.

Despite the requirements of PREPP there is no way of ensuring that nurses will choose to enhance their informatics skills or knowledge or indeed access other subject areas through this medium. However, if the profession is to use informatics as a tool for both learning and clinical practice, there needs to be a re-evaluation at practitioner level to critically examine what underpinning skills, knowledge and changes in attitude are necessary in order to effectively utilize nursing informatics to the full.

SKILLS

In order to facilitate the inputting of client data the employer needs to provide the necessary equipment capable of sustaining the high usage encountered within the health-care setting. It is therefore necessary that practitioners have access to sufficient terminals close by and have the necessary technical support to ensure that the system functions at all times. Within the initial procurement process the organization needs to recognize the importance of ongoing technical and software support, which will be needed once the system is in operation. This has led to the creation of a specific role of a nursing-based coordinator to maintain support mechanisms in some areas. The success of this role, however, is dependent upon this person being a sufficiently knowledgeable individual who is able to initiate changes to the system on behalf of nursing practitioners and influence interdisciplinary team members with a vested interest in the acquisition of information within the organization. Such measures should be examined carefully and adequately resourced, and there needs to be a ongoing commitment to the venture on behalf of all those in the organization if it is to succeed.

The initial training for practitioners varies greatly both in intensity and length between organizations. The employer must provide adequate training for all practitioners expected to access the system, viewing it as an investment in staff and the subsequent quality of information. Initial training must cover basic inputting skills and enable staff to become proficient with the functions of the system. Time out of the practice area needs to be devoted to this purpose and employers need to recognize the importance of further training if updates to the system are made. At this juncture an insightful employer will adopt a more educational approach and incorporate elements of the purpose of nursing informatics and data usage. Increased motivation is likely to arise if practitioners are made more aware of the importance and purpose of the data that they collect. This move towards education rather than training will promote ownership of the system through understanding and is more likely to ensure commitment on behalf of practitioners.

It is vital that employers recognize that, in order for a system to operate effectively, sufficient competent staff are required. It is simply not enough to train a few staff and expect them to be responsible for all the data entry within that area: this will lead to hostility from practitioners who picture themselves constantly attached to a computer terminal. An expectation that specific practitioners within the practice area can be relied upon for the cascading of informatics skills in the absence of formalized staff training is unsatisfactory. The nursing skill mix within the organization needs to reflect the commitment to information management. The tendencies to allow nursing aids to input nursing data and to provide non-permanent staff to bolster a dilute skill mix must be strongly resisted by both nursing managers and practitioners. If this is allowed to occur in practice it indicates a lack of insight on behalf of those involved as to the legal and professional implications that can arise.

The practitioner also needs to have guidelines as to what data and information are required by the employer. Alternative methods of data capture should be in place in case the system goes down. As local and national requirements alter, practitioners need to be informed. Methods such as user groups, on-screen information and updated reference materials on systems use can help to successfully disseminate this information. A local information strategy should incorporate all of these components as well as including further information on education and training.

Practitioners and employers need to develop evaluation skills to objectively examine what is currently elicited from nursing data and extract other pertinent areas of factual information that impact upon client care. Evaluation of care plans and the care provided by others within the interdisciplinary team presents the practitioner with access to reference material that influences research and evidence-based care. The organization, if there is a commitment to improving client care, will enable this interrogation of system databases by practitioners for research and clinical audit purposes. The impetus must come from practitioners to encourage professional development by making use of information that, albeit sensitive, is vital in the competitive market.

The level of informatics skill that each practitioner demonstrates in order to extract and use information meaningfully will undoubtedly vary. This may be because of his/her amount of exposure to the system, level of interest or confidence, expectation or insight as to what s/he can gain from the system. Those users with higher-level access or a greater knowledge base will certainly be able to elicit more useful information. However, this implies that there is a degree of elitism within the field of informatics, demonstrated by individual practitioners accessing relevant nursing information. Perhaps nursing informatics merely highlights the culture that is already in existence within the profession, whereby an informed practitioner recognizes the need to continuously update knowledge, skills and his/her professional profile within the health-care setting.

INFORMATICS AND PREPP

The introduction of PREPP (UKCC, 1995) has caused concern among many practitioners as to how they are to meet their development needs. The traditional forms of professional updating, such as short courses and study days offered by a local educational institution, are still viewed as being the most appropriate by practitioners. With the general absence of local trust strategies and the apparent freedom to pursue lifelong learning within the PREPP structure there is great potential for practitioners to explore alternative modes of knowledge acquisition. Information technology offers nurses many alternatives to traditional forms of education but presently is undertaken by few. For some, this is in part due to a lack of access; also, informatics may be viewed as a training tool that is somehow divorced from education and, therefore, from valuable knowledge acquisition.

In order to alter this perception, a change of culture is needed across all branches of the profession. The value placed on learning needs to be re-evaluated by many professionals and the misconception that knowledge of worth is something only taught within a classroom should be dismissed. A reassessment of the delivery of education needs to be scrutinized by all those involved. Unless such processes are undertaken by the profession itself the desired outcomes of PREPP will only be met in part. The current trend of pressured staffing issues and alterations in educational funding indicate that future educational opportunities for practitioners will depend increasingly upon self-financing and devotion of a practitioner's own time for study. Nursing informatics offers a means of effective education that can be accessed when a practitioner requires, and the possibility of developing packages for large numbers of learners to ensure cost effectiveness.

RESOURCES

There are many technological, as well as more conventional sources to aid learning that can be drawn upon to increase nursing knowledge and improve practice. The practitioner can support learning of this nature at many levels and through a variety of means. Access to resources is dependent upon what is available in the practitioner's local environment, i.e. the personal, clinical or educational setting.

Computer-assisted learning

Within the educational or clinical setting there may be computer-assisted learning (CAL) software packages that can be accessed by practitioners. Such packages can be run in conjunction with a form of assessment, with accreditation being given upon successful completion of learning. This form of self-study is worthwhile in areas in which the practitioner should regularly update skills and knowledge, e.g. resuscitation, drug administration.

CD-ROM and CDI

The developments in compact disk technology have resulted in the creation of databases or libraries that are held on CD-ROM and CDI laser-read disks. Many that are now available contain reference and interactive material. The information that they contain can be used by the practitioner for personal professional updating and to reinforce skills such as resuscitation or moving and handling techniques. The use of CD-ROM or CDI in updating skills can be coupled with a formal or informal assessment while 'on-line', which can be accredited by organizations and contribute towards PREPP.

The majority of CD-ROMs used in practice are databases, or libraries of information, accessed by the practitioner for reference. The Royal College of Nursing bibliography and interactive anatomy and physiology CD-ROMs are published as an addition to the traditional text format.

Another source widely used by practitioners is the Cochrane Library. This consists of four main databases.

- **The Cochrane Database of Systematic Reviews (CDSR)** includes the full text of the regularly updated systematic reviews of the effects of health care prepared by the Cochrane Collaboration.
- **The Database of Abstracts of Reviews of Effectiveness (DARE)** is prepared by the National Health Service Centre for Reviews and Dissemination at the University of York. This database provides information on previously published reviews of the effects of health care.
- **The Cochrane Controlled Trials Register (CCTR)** comprises records that have been identified as reports of definite or possible randomized or quasi-randomized trials, primarily through hand-searching of journals within the Cochrane Collaboration.
- **The Cochrane Review Methodology Database** consists of a bibliography intended to help those who are new to the science of reviewing to find additional material of interest, and those who are already immersed in it to find something new.

As with all contemporary reference material it is important that sources are updated. Many publishers of databases offer a service of forwarding revised compact disks by subscription.

Local nursing systems

The vision for nursing within the NHS has been to incorporate the use of informatics into everyday practice (NHSME, 1994). However, in practice the level of access to information systems and indeed the versatility of systems varies greatly. Hospital information support systems have the potential in most instances to support databases and library information to aid the practitioner with both informed patient care, and extending professional knowledge and research activities.

In practice, nursing systems may function as part of a network or exist as a stand-alone system such as a PC. The software used on the system also has a bearing on the types of function that the practitioner can realistically expect. Many computer-assisted packages and databases rely upon Microsoft Windows and therefore will not function on systems that are DOS-only. The inclusion of a CD-ROM drive is rarely found on networked systems used within the NHS environment at present, but many stand-alone PCs 'secreted' within the organization have this facility.

The Internet

This is a large, complex international computer network, which holds a vast array and quantity of data accessed via a telephone link. The Internet allows users to access publicly available files, e-mail, discussion groups and the WorldWide Web

(WWW), which consists of numerous pages of information, many of which are interactive.

Useful Internet addresses

There are a range of helpful sites relating to organizations, information pages, departments and search engines. It is important to be aware that addresses may change as sites are updated. Current journals and publications can often be accessed via the Internet, their addresses being printed in the text version. The list below illustrates a few examples of Internet addresses: however, on the WWW the choice is seemingly inexhaustible.

- Achoo (health search engine): http://www.achoo.com/
- Department of Health: http://www.open.gov.uk/doh
- English National Board: http://www.enb.org.uk/
- MEDLINE: http://www.healthgate.com
- NURSENET website (discussion group):
  http://www.ualberta.ca/~jrnorris/nursenet/nn.html
- Office of Data Protection: http://www.open.gov.uk/dpr/dprhome.htm
- Rod Ward's on-line resource list: http://www.shef.ac.uk/~nhcon/

COMPUTER-MEDIATED ENVIRONMENTS

Computer-mediated communication (CMC)

CMC is currently being used and has the potential for further expansion in a number of areas, including professional contact, continuing professional education and clinical support. The practitioner can access such areas via CMC by e-mail, computer conferencing, discussion lists and special interest groups.

Advances in computer and communications technology, recent development and awareness of the Internet have all contributed to CMC uptake increasing momentum. In nursing, this is still in its infancy but there is an increasing awareness of the great potential of this medium.

In practice, the opportunities that CMC offers practitioners include access to ideas, information, discussion and debates. From this, practitioners can reflect individually or work collaboratively with others from their own discipline or from a multiprofessional perspective at national or international level. While this individual approach supports updating of knowledge and an environment for the cross-fertilization of ideas, it could also be developed into a system that provides direct clinical support for practitioners, patients and carers within community areas.

Within the sphere of continuing professional education this approach lends itself to practitioners who undertake ongoing study in their own time or those who geographically are unable to access appropriate courses locally.

Applied computer-mediated study

On-line courses offering distance learning have recently been developed and offer the practitioner an alternative way to engage in continuing professional education, mainly at postgraduate level.

One example of this mode of study is currently facilitated by the University of Greenwich, this unique, innovative programme being the MSc in Continuing Professional Development (Health) (Collaborative Learning Through Reflective Practice and Computer Mediated Communication). The programme is supported by a number of underpinning concepts. These include continuing professional development, reflective practice, collaborative learning and critical thinking. Such concepts are essential components for the furthering of nursing knowledge and practice, mirroring the philosophy of PREPP but within a multiprofessional environment.

It could indeed be argued that such components could constitute a more traditionally taught course at master's level. However, it is both the process and approach that make this course unique. The distance learning facilitation style and the use of CMC through computer conferencing and e-mail has transformed the traditional modes of learning into a potentially new paradigm (Jordan and Ryan, 1997). It engages students in group activities, promoting learner interaction with peers, which is actively supported by teacher input.

The concept of CMC acknowledges the value of the adult learner within the learning environment and views them as a very rich resource (Knowles, 1990). This can be because the students are experienced practitioners, as well as the way in which the CMC system captures the content of the virtual classroom interactions and archives them for reflection at a later date.

An example of the student experience would include tutor-devised structured activities in which they are required to discuss and debate within a conference environment contained within a virtual classroom. Students are also required to work collaboratively in smaller groups. The environment is asynchronous in nature, which gives students time to reflect, apply critical thinking and give a considered response, thus facilitating a deeper level of learning.

The multiprofessional environment experienced by these students promotes effective communication and collaboration. This encourages critical thinking, discussion and debate pertaining to clinical practice, moving them away from insular professional practice and often purely local ideas to a national or international multidisciplinary perspective. Such anticipated changes in thinking mirror what is being professionally promoted and aimed at by nursing practitioners in relation to the long-term objectives of PREPP and the concept of the lifelong learner (ENB, 1994). Such aims are achieved by sharing professional knowledge and analysing how our own practice relates to or reflects that of other professionals and how it will underpin future evidence-based improvements in nursing practice.

REFERENCES

ENB (1994) *Creating Lifelong Learners – Partnerships for Care*, English National Board for Nursing, Midwifery and Health Visiting, London

ENB (1995) *Creating Lifelong Learners*, English National Board for Nursing, Midwifery and Health Visiting, London.

Jordan, G. G. and Ryan, M. (1997) Computer-mediated communication (CMC) – a collaborative tool for continuing professional development (CPD), in *Super Highways, Super CAL, Super Learning – CAL '97 International Conference Proceedings, Exeter, March 1997*, (ed. L. Baggott), COTE, University of Exeter, Exeter.

Knowles, M. (1990) *The Adult Learner: a Neglected Species*, 4th edn, Gulf Publishing, Houston, TX.

Leeder, T. (1991), cited by King, W. (1994) The need for information requirements analysis and evaluation, in *Nursing Informatics*, (ed. P. Wainwright), Churchill Livingstone, Edinburgh.

NHSME (1992) *IM & T Strategy Overview*, NHS Management Executive, Bristol.

NHSME (1994) *Information Systems for Nurses, Midwives and Health Visitors – A strategic statement*, NHS Management Executive (Information Management Group), Leeds.

Office for Data Protection (1984) Data Protection Act 1984, HMSO, London.

UKCC (1993) *Standards for Records and Record Keeping*, United Kingdom Central Council for Nursing, Midwifery and Health Visiting, London.

UKCC (1995) *PREP*, United Kingdom Central Council for Nursing, Midwifery and Health Visiting, London.

UKCC (1996) *Guidelines for Professional Practice*, United Kingdom Central Council for Nursing, Midwifery and Health Visiting, London.

Index